Information Technology and Contemporary Healthcare Issues

George O. Obikoya

Table of Content

Executive Summary

Healthcare delivery in the C21st is going to be increasingly different from what it used to be for a number of reasons, chief among which is the increasing realization of the need for health services to conform to the basic economic principles to which other sectors of the economy conform. This would be necessary because of the likely increasing scarcity of healthcare resources and the need to optimize resource allocation and utilization. Yet, health jurisdictions worldwide would face equally profound pressures from healthcare consumers to improve the quality of healthcare delivery, and to make it more accessible, and more affordable. These twin pressures on health jurisdictions would necessitate the rethinking of all aspects of healthcare delivery, the need for them in particular to pursue vigorously the achievement of the dual healthcare delivery objectives of delivering high quality healthcare simultaneously reducing health spending.

It would be evident to all stakeholders that it is only intuitive for health systems and indeed, all stakeholders to attempt to achieve these goals. This would be more so as the intricate link between their health and their fortunes would also become clearer, their health connected inescapably with the economy of their countries. Setting goals, therefore, which would ensure that they receive qualitative healthcare, but not deplete their wallets or the wealth of their countries, compromising their ability, and that of their countries to have sufficient resources left to engage in other important activities would no doubt receive the appropriate acclamation.

The path toward achieving the dual healthcare delivery objectives would nonetheless, be tortuous. It would require health jurisdictions and systems to identify and address key issues that have both health and non-health roots, but are crucial to the numerous processes involved in the healthcare delivery enterprise to reach their respective goals, all of which eventually result in the delivery of services at the point of care to a particular healthcare consumer. We will examine some of such issues in this e-book, with a view to better understanding them, vis-à-vis their roles in contemporary healthcare delivery and how we could improve which latter manipulating them, in our quest to achieve the dual healthcare delivery objectives.

Introduction

The new healthcare delivery dispensation would feature ideas in both the

health and nonhealth domains emerging at a rapid pace, instigating changes in health services delivery that would compel not just health systems, but individual healthcare consumers to embrace the dual healthcare delivery objectives of qualitative health services delivery simultaneously reducing health spending. Progress in medical knowledge for example would certainly necessitate changes in the way we practice medicine, and even spawn new models of healthcare delivery. Developments in healthcare information and communication technologies would also offer new approaches to facilitating the many processes involved in healthcare delivery, helping to reduce transactions costs, hence health spending, while improving the quality of care delivered. The two domains would likely feed into each other, one helping to improve the other, both ensuring progress toward the achievement of the dual healthcare delivery goals.

As healthcare delivery could never be perfect, due to the disruptive effects of

those forces, inherent in health systems and external to them, operating and triggering changes that the health systems must inevitably undergo, the onus would be on all healthcare stakeholders to act to ensure the achievement of the dual healthcare delivery goals. We will explore the issues, problems, and challenges in the way of achieving these objectives, and in the process reveal some of the measures applicable to overcoming them, and to moving on relentlessly towards the achievement of these important goals. That we cannot afford to ignore healthcare delivery, regardless of our health jurisdiction, and its funding system, for example, is no longer in doubt, as not only would we not be meeting the most fundamental mandate of such systems of providing qualitative healthcare to all, the funds would dry up anyway. Even before it does, if it ever got to that stage, we would have little choice but to confront these issues and resolve them, as pressures mount, from all quarters for health systems to justify their very existence. Addressing and overcoming the challenges that confront health systems and change them remarkably, down the road would be endeavors we would owe to ourselves, and the generations of individuals coming after us.

Is a long-term care crisis imminent in developed countries?

The prevention and reduction of requirements for long-term care (LTC), services and supports an individual needs when aging, chronic illnesses, or disability has compromised the ability to care for oneself, is a key goal of the long-term care insurance system in Japan, yet the certified care levels of most care-recipients have depreciated since the system's implementation in 2000[1]. Demands for services at facilities instead of in-home services are on the rise, waiting lists for public nursing homes are longer than ever, and the rates of residential care in for-profit private homes is fast increasing, with out-of-pocket costs implications, the system, essentially of minimal benefit to many individuals in the country. Five years on, the high public anticipation of the change in April 2006 in the insurance system is understandable and preventive care is a key aspect of the change expected to help reduce the cost of care services[2] that care workers in the community would provide over a million people with supportive care needs, ushering a new era of LTC. The new comprehensive community health centers built would facilitate service provision, including evaluation for preventive care, and consultations for families and caregivers, each prefecture expected to undertake continuous quality assessment, with the results made public via the Internet and other media, to enable informed decision-making on the choice of care provision and or providers. The likely extensive potential involvement of healthcare information and communication technologies in the many initiatives that the success of the new scheme would warrant is evident. The government's new system of community based services for examples group homes, small and multifunctional care services, and day care services for people with dementia will add to the service mix evolving in the reform efforts underway in the long-term care domain in the country. Will these changes be sufficient to avert a potential crisis in long-term care in the country, the worsening status of which had deepened to the point where homicides of disabled seniors by their burnt-out caregivers remain prevalent[1]? Many in Japan would think not, and would be unlikely to consider any measure short of overhauling the entire health system adequate. Dissatisfaction with long-term care is not peculiar to Japan, but is in fact, typical of the situation in many developed countries, where LTC on the one hand is a reality for millions of fragile seniors, a source of immense angst for many more[3], and their relatives. What is more, many in these countries view their governments' LTC policies as flawed, with seniors themselves paying an ever-higher portion of their healthcare costs. Yet, the increasing population of the elderly with implications for dire economic projections makes it inevitable for these governments to view

LTC issues with the clarity of insight coupled with an objective yet suave consideration of the increasing political pressure by seniors in these countries for change on these issues, in prescribing solutions to them. For these and many other reasons some in fact rooted in what the unwary might deem unrelated to these issues if not even irrelevant, few if any governments in these countries can afford to ignore the issues concerning LTC, in particular its financing, or indeed, the need to address them urgently, considering the projected increase in the need for LTC. In the U.S., for example, experts may not concur on the future rates of disabilities among seniors in the country, but even if they did not change from their current values, the country would still have more persons with long-term care needs. Indeed, that the population of those in the 85 years and above group, the likeliest to do so, projected according to U.S. Census Bureau, 2004 estimates, to double between 2000-2030 and even quadruple by 2050, makes the urgency that the attention these issues require even starker. Is it any wonder then in this context that some want the healthcare costs implications factored in health systems where healthcare is free, with seniors' money transitioning to heirs, widening the wealth difference between rich, who have inheritances and the financially challenged? On the other hand, should we discountenance the ethico-moral roots of the decision in Scotland to jettison the distinction made between personal and nursing care and providing seniors, personal care gratis who need it? Should we in fact be making the distinction between personal and nursing care in the case of seniors at least when several studies indicate that most residents of all varieties of care homes have dementia, which makes it meaningless essentially to group care homes into residential and nursing homes[4]? Should we not be focusing on providing these seniors with care tailored to the needs of persons with dementia, specifically specialist dementia care? Yet, is there room for such arguments as viewing life's full cycle in its splendor and perpetual value until death, and even beyond, as opposed to an increasingly disposable baggage best left to wither, relic of an amortized appliance-swap mindset? Could we integrate these concerns with those of the funding requirements for assuring the delivery of qualitative long term care to our seniors and others in society for examples those with some form of mental and physical disabilities and those without the financial wherewithal to fund such care but need them? Many consider one of the major flaws of Japan's mandatory long-term-care social insurance system mentioned earlier as not recognizing the significance of considering dementia in LTC planning and budgeting, the activities of daily living (ADL)-based evaluations misclassifying many with Alzheimer's able to feed and dress themselves in lower-needs categories. Besides these individuals, not receiving required services, even when appropriately classified, the services available were mostly for rather intensive care, calculated in minutes, when in fact persons with dementia should have the exact opposite sort of care, benign, unhurried care estimated in hours. Do we not in fact need a rethinking of the entire concept of long-term care in keeping with the realities of our times and projections of the status down the road? Let us consider one important dimension of the LTC issue. Relatives and friends often provide LTC at home, and some individuals obtain the services via home and community-based services, for examples home health or personal care, and adult day care, or in institutions, for examples residential care or nursing homes. The emphasis that each country or health jurisdiction places on each of these sources of LTC varies. In Japan for example, relatively inexpensive Alzheimer's group homes are gaining currency, considered residences and not institutions, on the Scandinavian model. In the U.S., individuals with long-term care needs in the Medicaid program include those with mental illness, mental retardation and developmental disabilities, spinal cord and traumatic brain injuries, Alzheimer's disease and other dementias, and those with neurodegenerative diseases, and children with special care needs. Most persons with LTC needs in the U.S for example live in the community, about 80% of all care to persons with LTC needs living in the community provided by their relatives and friends, a very small percentage depending solely on paid support. With the country currently having no national system of long-term care insurance, and people essentially depending on their own funds first and then chiefly on Medicaid, the latter the primary payer LTC services particularly nursing home care, but for which many in fact do not meet the eligibility criteria, would many not end up excluded from needed LTC? To compound these issues many of these individuals often also lack the financial resources or have insufficient amounts to meet the costs of their often chronic and multiple health conditions, which in particular renders any consideration of the typically expensive private sector services redundant. Families and friends for example, resort to paid services using mostly their own funds, when no longer able to care for the person requiring LTC, this sometimes so because there is no relative available to give the care, or the intensity of care has become overwhelming psychologically and perhaps physically. Yet, personal care and nursing home care costs on the yearly average hover around $10,000 and $75,000 respectively. Does the country therefore not need urgent policy options to address increasing requirements for LTC and the associated costs and other issues? To be sure, Medicare and some private LTC insurance also pay for LTC in the U.S., but with even Medicare about to start to pay for services out of its trust fund that a thorough review of LTC funding and the establishment of newer and more appropriate policies in the country is crucial is not in doubt. Despite that spending via Medicare, the federal health insurance program for seniors and persons less than 65 years with lasting disabilities, on LTC is restricted, and relatives and friends fund most LTC expenses, the U.S. still spent more than $150 billion in 2003 on LTC, mostly on nursing home care. Nonetheless, the question about Medicare covering all LTC needs is not controversial, as it does not, paying only for some categories of LTC such as for home health services to recipients unable to leave home, that require part-time expert nursing/therapy services, and treated by a doctor, and limited nursing home care, for a hundred days, for post-acute care persons. Medicaid also has eligibility restrictions, to qualify requiring being poor, although have limited assets for example savings accounts, and being over 65 years old or disabled. Are the numbers of individuals for who these restrictions would make receiving LTC difficult if not impossible likely to increase with population aging, and could an LTC crisis in fact be looming?

A recent report by the Joseph Rowntree Foundation highlighting the need for

an overhaul of the funding arrangements for the long term care of elderly people echoes this concern regarding the United Kingdom, and underscores the fact that concerns about a potential crisis in long-term care is not peculiar to the U.S[5]. The report noted that if the country did not, it would confront a major shortfall in care as the population ages in the forthcoming decades. According to the report, the U.K is yet to find a clear, fair, and adequate system for financing the increasing demand for LTC, having as the report stressed "shied away from major reform" in the 1990s during which period, other countries for examples, Japan and Germany were reforming their systems. Commenting on the report, Christopher Kelly, former permanent secretary at the Department of Health said, "If we continue with this already overstretched, inequitable, and incomprehensible system of funding while demand continues to rise, there will be serious costs for the dignity and wellbeing of older people". Figures recently published by Eurostat indicate that European Union (EU) member states spend more each year to fund the costs of old age, sickness, unemployment, housing and children, 28%, 27.4% and 26.9% of their GDP on social benefits in 2003, 2002, and 2000 respectively. The 25 EU countries seem in fact to be moving closer to the 1993 values, when the EU's 15 member states spent 28.7% of GDP on social benefits[6]. Even then, the 15 'old' member states spend on average about 10% more of their GDP on their social systems than the ten new members, the spending expressed as percentage of GDP, the differences even more expressed in Purchasing Power Standards (PPS), which factors in cross-border purchasing-price differences. Significantly, the figures also show that high spending on social welfare is not necessarily harmful to a country's economic well-being, the EU's most competitive countries namely Denmark, Finland, Ireland, Sweden and the UK all in the top ten regarding the percentage of their GDP spent on social protection. In fact, the figures also show that the Baltic countries, where poverty is among highest in the EU, are in the bottom positions, which put together the figures seem to suggest that investment in social cohesion is a key asset for boosting a country's competitiveness and economic development. Does this argument not extend to the health domain including to long-term care? Would investing in LTC not on the one hand ease the financial and psychological burden on the families and relatives involved in the care of affected persons needing LTC, and on the other those on society at large, the provision of qualitative care to these individuals reducing overall costs of care ultimately? In other words, caring for those needing long-term care is not just a moral obligation of society, considering not just the perspective of human dignity, but also the contributions they have made to societal progress one way or another, even by their very presence being here giving some people joy. Indeed, many also continue to make such contributions or have the potential so to do. Furthermore, do these considerations also not have the potential to contribute to a country's economic development? With the imminent increase in the numbers of persons that will need such care, should we not in fact be considering ways by which we could improve the quality of care that these individuals receive while simultaneously reducing associated costs? As with other domains of healthcare delivery, long-term care is a multiplicity of transactions, whose costs if not curtailed could be quite substantial. Should there not be therefore serious considerations on how to reduce these transactions costs? What role could the implementation and use of the appropriate healthcare information and communication technologies play in this regard? Would the effective monitoring for example of the health status of an individual in a nursing home that suffers from a chronic illness remotely help reduce the prospects of complications of the disease whose management would for example require the persons transferred to the hospital with costs implications for the stay and prescription medications, not to mention diagnostic investigations? How much money could we save implementing such technologies in the management of the possibly millions of individuals that might have such chronic diseases? Even investing in such technologies that could prevent falls in the elderly for example could save many the emotional and financial burden associated with the treatment of bone fractures, in effect, we would not just be reducing costs but be delivering qualitative long-term care at the same time. In other words we would be achieving the dual healthcare delivery objectives (DHDO) that are crucial to meeting the challenges of contemporary and future healthcare delivery overall. There is no doubt that the projections of the amount many countries in the developed world would spend on domiciliary and institutional long term care are dire, according to some experts, 10.8% of it gross national product (GNP) by the U.K., for example by 2030[7], without intervention to ensure the achievement of such goals as the DHDO mentioned above. As with most other developed countries Norway expects to a significant ageing of its population in the years ahead, perhaps less dramatically compared to other Organization for Economic Cooperation and Development (OECD) countries[8]. The proportion of those 65 or older will increase from about 15% of the population to 23% by 2040, the old-age dependency ratio, those 65 and older relative to those of working age, billed to rise from 26% to 43 per cent by 2040, versus over 50% per cent for the OECD. The number of people of working age per old-age person will therefore decrease, from 4 to 2.3[8]. With its employment rates of seniors among the highest in the OECD, pension outlays relatively low and substantial financial assets piled away in the Government Petroleum Fund, the cushioning of the effects of population ageing on its economy is not be very surprising if at all. Nonetheless, even Norway needs reforms as with its pension system maturing ageing would result in one of the largest increases in pension spending as a share of GDP in OECD countries over the next five decades, with potential adverse implications fro long-term care in the country. With the fiscal impact of ageing expected to manifest in a projected doubling of the cost of the country's pension system, and health care spending for the elderly expected to increase substantially, Norway should doubtless start now if not already to examine ways by which it would reduce the costs of healthcare delivery, including long-term care. It should in fact be seeking ways to improve simultaneously the quality of its health services, including investing in that healthcare information and communication technologies at different healthcare delivery levels that have the potential to enable and facilitate its achievement of these dual healthcare delivery goals. Again, other countries in the developed world would also need to take similar measures most appropriate to the contexts in which they deliver care. As earlier stated, and in general these countries would need to examine the transactions involved in long-term care, and thoroughly too. They would in fact also need to redefine the concepts of long-term care including for example eschewing ageism. They would need to have a clear idea of the need for objectivity in their approach to these issues rather than bogging down the discourse with outmoded prejudices that might even be detrimental to their abilities to address the multifarious issues that population aging would spawn in the coming years. Examples of such issues include the potential need to reconsider retirement age, with a view to extending it, and for pensions' reforms. In re-examining the conceptual roots of long-term care for example, it would be necessary also as earlier stated to consider the pivotal position of Alzheimer's disease and the other dementias in resource allocation and utilization. They also need to revisit the theoretical issues regarding other important conditions for which some individuals might require long-term care for examples mental retardation, and traumatic brain disorders, with a view to determining the appropriate care levels and the milieu best suited for its delivery. The fundamental reasons for these re-conceptualizations is to facilitate the adjustments of service provision required to meet the demands of changing times, for example, the most effective approaches to service provision based on changes in employment/unemployment rates. These are issues not only critical in all countries considering population aging, and the declining birth rates in many developed countries, but more so in countries in which illegal immigration is a key issue such as the U.S, and in those in which membership of regional bodies for example the EU is changing the dynamics of immigration. The inflow of a variety of professional cadres, and the approaches to remuneration for them, including the incentives to work in the variety of community-based initiatives that constitute important elements of long-term care, are for examples important considerations in this regard. So are the knowledge of this workforce and the interests of the individual workers in for example, the use of healthcare information and communication technologies (ICT), technologies that would feature prominently increasingly in long-term care provision, among others, in the near future. These considerations are also essential elements of any efforts to curtail the transactions costs of the activities involved in long-term care delivery. Thus for example in delineating the functionalities such as being able to carry out one's activities of daily living (ADL), and others germane to our new concepts of long-term care, our recruitment and retention efforts would be more focused, as would service provision. This focus would be even more valuable for example, with the efforts coupled with projected statistics of the numbers of persons for whom long-term care would be necessary, among other characterizations. Thus, we should be working toward making long-term care provision as effective and efficient as possible, for example, avoiding costly policy flaws as having persons receiving domiciliary care costing $800 per week in a locality where residential care is available for $200, capping domiciliary care spending at about the cost of institutional care[9].

The point here is that a fundamental rethinking of long-term care is the first

thing we need to do to avert the potential crisis in the developed world due to a number of factors including population aging and the equally significant healthcare and social welfare funding issues that confront these countries and would likely be worse in the years ahead. With regard the funding scarcity in the face of increasing health spending that they experience, measures taken to solve this problem, for example investing in healthcare ICT, with its potential to help in the achievement of the DHDO, could no doubt also help in averting any long-term care crisis. Such measures, deployed for example, in primary disease prevention, or even in the prompt and accurate diagnosis and treatment of diseases, or secondary disease prevention, could help minimize disability hence reduce the need for care, including long-term care in later life. This would the establishment of initiatives toward healthy aging, an important starting point in these countries, in efforts geared toward achieving such goals. There is no doubt about the potential role that healthcare ICT would play in actualizing such initiatives in particular in countries where not only are many seniors computer literate, but also where there are increasing numbers of sophisticated multimedia opportunities for reaching them. The financial outlays of such initiatives would no doubt constitute aspects of the health spending that these countries want to reduce. However, the benefits that would accrue in the long term from these investments in terms of improved health hence declining healthcare costs and in those of the emotional and other disease burden in general, would likely far outweigh the investments. Thus in considering another important measure we need to take to avert any future long-term care crisis, that of curtailing spending, and indeed, of how to fund the imminent increase in long-term care needs in the first place, we need to acknowledge the likely need for some initial spending whose benefits we would later reap in many important respects. Concerning our funding options, we also need to acknowledge the need to ease the soaring out-of-pocket expenses individuals requiring LTC and their families and friends incur now, which as we have noted could be quite significant, individually and on the aggregate. This is considering also that in countries such as in the U.S., they are responsible for the bulk of the expenses for these services, directly, and in countries, for example in the U.K., also albeit essentially indirectly via taxes among others. This latter, is why some query the value of insurance as a source of funding for long-term care in countries such as the U.K., except perhaps for the well heeled, or at taxpayer's expense, for the not-so-financially-endowed. Even in countries such as the U.S., private long-term care could be pricey, in particular for the poor the average base premium for a 65 year old was $1,337 per year in 2002, just 9 million policies sold, just over 6 million in force as also policy terminations often follow default in premium payments, likelier with retired seniors. Further, premiums become more costly the older the applicant is, hence for most of the people who would likely need long-term care, if they did not buy the insurance earlier in life. What is more, coverage is typically restricted, although most private long-term care insurance plans cover assisted living facilities, home health care, nursing homes, hospices and respite care, some also, others for examples, caregiver training, homemaker/chore services, and case management services. Efforts to encourage more individuals to purchase private LTC insurance have resulted in sales growth although not significantly. Indeed, with many of the opinion that they do not really aid those that need them and do not seem to be keen on younger persons with disabilities, among other issues, that the adoption of private long-term care insurance in the country would become increasingly widespread could only be conjectural. With regard taxes, many regard the hypothecated tax for long-term care introduced in Germany in the early 1990s merely replaced a liability applying on families, which no doubt would have caused consternation among working families in some other European countries asked to pay taxes to protect the inheritances of richer people, a non-selective inheritance tax more acceptable. The contribution to the national insurance scheme (NIS) in Norway is low versus the standard rate for employees and persons receiving a minimum pension pay no contribution whatsoever. Furthermore, pensioners receive a higher basic deduction and in some cases, could benefit from special limitations on tax, all favorable tax regulations that make retirement essentially more inexpensive, than in most other OECD countries hence besides the disincentives in the country's old-age pensions scheme to continue to work after the age 67 years , strengthen the incentives for early retirement. These examples illustrate some of the issues that we need to examine in our new more inclusive approach to conceptualizing long-term care funding. For how long should individuals keep working for example? Should we institute measures, rules, even policies that would make it unattractive to retire early or that, would promote working past current retirement age, and should we extend that age? Would we be reducing the chances of individuals developing illnesses staying at home doing nothing that could result in their ending up in long-term care facilities? In other words, could working longer be contributory to the reduction in morbidities that would reduce long-term care service utilization thus overall health spending? There is a surfeit of literature on the beneficial effects of physical exercise, which going to work might be the key source of for an elderly person working past current retirement age. It might also be the only opportunity for some of these individuals to socialize and not be lonely and miserable having lost their spouses perhaps siblings and friends to death, hence saved the agony of depression and possibly suicide, common in seniors that live alone. Should we therefore subscribe to the contention by some of the justifiability of diverting resources away from the elderly[10] or embrace that by others that not only does ageing not cause disease, but also that regular physical activity in the senior years could 'rejuvenate' physical capacity by 10-15 years[11]? Research studies have shown that regular physical activity reduces the risk of coronary heart disease, diabetes, colon cancer, and several other chronic diseases. It is perhaps easier to convince individuals about the health benefits of exercise, which is a subset of physical activity, defined as planned, structured, repetitive movement performed with the aim of improving/maintaining physical fitness than to be merely active physically. This is why going to work, the stipend accruable from which is persuasion enough, could be significant, especially for seniors, who might in fact be reluctant to engage in exercises for fear of damage to their health for example. However, with the increasing novelties of computer-generated exercise modules delivered via a variety of multimedia portals, and capable of use with no health risks by seniors in the comfort of their homes, should we not in fact be promoting with vigor, the idea of healthy ageing and encouraging seniors to purchase these technologies for example? No doubt, the prevalence of cardiovascular diseases is higher in old age, but this does mean aging causes these diseases nor that they are inevitable in old age. Should we therefore not, as part of our re-conceptualization of long-term care start to emphasize besides how best to care for those that need it, also how to reduce the prevalence of illness and disability in old age and promote healthier aging? By so doing, we would be deferring so to speak, the onset of disability in our seniors, which would result in a healthier older population, who would therefore benefit from a shorter period of dependency prior to death. This means less use of long-term care and less costs incurred from these services, hence less spending on them, and overall on healthcare delivery, of course without having done anything to compromise healthcare delivery to both seniors and all, and in fact, having improved the quality of service delivery simultaneously. These are achievable goals that health systems worldwide and in particular in developed countries would have to pursue inevitably as the new realities of healthcare delivery dawn on them, literally. In other words rather than health promotion among the elderly and longevity meaning an increase in the number of years spent in chronic disability, we ensure that they mean happy and productive years to family, friends, and society, and a shorter period of dependency before death. It is clear from the foregoing that we need to begin to rethink several aspects of long-term care, with a view to modifying our approaches to addressing the issues involved, more so considering the projected increase in the numbers of baby-boomers that would soon retire, and the ongoing population ageing in the developed world in particular. Both of these events and others would no doubt have significant costs implication for health and social services delivery hence warrant pre-emptive attention. Still on funding long-term care therefore, we must continue to seek potential and real options, for example, the costs of most long-term care being part of the social services budget, an aspect of a strategy offering an approach to diffusing and bankrolling costs. However, a variant of this approach that surfaced in the U.K in the mid-1990s some considered simply liquidating the assets of the elderly to the betterment of nursing home shareholders, a selective heritage tax from which in addition the seniors might benefit little if at all. Developments in the pension domain attest to the intercalation of factors and the complexity of the issue of long-term care, and of health in general. In the U.S., some states and local governments are starting to question the guarantees protecting government workers' pensions, guarantees often supported by union contracts, and protecting over 15 million individuals, and which many believe are even stronger than those on pensions in the private sector are. The questioning predicates on what to do about an over $2 trillion debt in unfunded retirement benefits and retiree health plans obligations by state and local governments for their workers[11]. A new Governmental Accounting Standards Board rule due to commence operations in 2007, would likely find out the true extent of the debt, the retiree health benefits alone estimated to be about $1.4 trillion[11], and impel the reforms that many hope would obviate the potential tax hikes future generations might have to endure, as baby boomers retire en masse. Such tax hikes would have adverse implications for competitiveness and job losses. Experts have suggested the need for slashing benefits, and initiating pre-funded savings-based pension plans, as Alaska and Michigan have started with their new employees, contribution to the saving account stipulated, the former also, a health-care plan, high-deductible insurance and a Health Savings Account (HSA) included. Coupled with cutting retirement benefits, in particular for younger employees, increased significantly in the 1990s, state and local governments expending on the average, $3.91 per hour worked on employee health benefits, versus the private sector's $1.72, some consider necessary for averting the likelihood of the fiscal crisis[11]. There is no doubt that these guarantees help secure seniors' financial buoyancy in retirement, which could be crucial to their abilities to fund long-term care if ever required. Yet, not only could government's huge indebtedness compromise its potential contribution to long-term care, via Medicare and Medicaid, for examples, its deciding to solve the problem by increasing taxes could compromise the country's economic buoyancy. This could make it even more difficult to fund long-term triggering a slippery slope so to say that could have potential ramifications in all aspects of the country's life. Thus, reduced competitiveness in the industries could compromise employment status, with many out of jobs adversely affecting psychological and in turn physical health of the individuals involved, and possibly their families, further putting pressure on the health system. Thus, we need to devise a means whereby those requiring funds for long-term care, for examples, seniors, would be able to afford hence access such care without creating economic chaos in the country.

The search for ways to finance long-term care therefore continues and needs

to be all-inclusive. How for example, could we make long-term care less costly and yet more qualitative? This dual healthcare delivery objectives (DHDO) in fact applies to not just long-term care, but also to healthcare delivery in general. Even if it involves upfront investments in healthcare information and communication technologies (ICT) for example, technologies that have the potential to help achieve the DHDO, would the benefits accruable from this investment, even if in the long term, not outweigh the pecuniary setback due to the amount invested in the first place? The use of these technologies might in fact be in aspects of care delivery immediately remote from the clinical domain, yet still be crucial to the achievement overall of the DHDO. In other words, as with healthcare delivery in general, we need to start to view long-term care in a more global way, recognizing the importance of all the processes involved in achieving the delivery of long-term care. We should also recognize the need to make the processes more efficient and effective, as critical aspects of our efforts to finance LTC successfully, hence ensure it fulfills its promise. Medicare and private health plans for example are increasingly 'mining' claims data for potential fraud with the help of cutting-edge computer technology[12]. There is no doubt that this would help significantly to reduce fraud, which accounts between 3% and 10% of the $2 trillion spent annually on health care in the U.S., whose impact on long-term care would equally doubtless be significant. IBM, ViPS, Fair Isaac, and a UnitedHealth Group subsidiary, Ingenix, among other firms, have recently been developing software able to detect via 'spider-webbing,' suspicious claims data patterns. Red flags pointing toward possible fraud include uncompetitive pricing by healthcare providers, for example charging above what their peers charge; healthcare providers ordering more tests/procedures per patient than do their peers, or those that carry out medically 'unlikely' procedures. Others include healthcare providers that bill for more expensive procedures and equipment when less expensive options are available, and patients that travel long distances to receive treatment. These technologies are actually yielding dividends, Aetna's, helping the insurer foil over $89 million in fraudulent reimbursements in 2005 versus $15 million it recouped after making fraudulent payments. Would the company not consider its investment in this software worthwhile after all? Indeed, such software enables firms to save much more money by detecting fraud prior to claims payments than recovering the money afterward as it does state and federal governments. The South Carolina Department of Health and Human Services for example recently implemented its Medicaid anti-fraud program, between then, August 2005, and October 2006 the agency, which also implemented the software to help in overall optimal resource management has started already to reap financial gains. Thus, the software also enables the agency to make such important decision as those regarding the cost-effectiveness of medical procedures, for example, the effectiveness or otherwise of certain screening exercises, in disease prevention. This is in addition to the software revealing cryptic event s such as double billing for physician consultation by Medicaid patients that are under an all-inclusive billing rate, for example, with a potential $1 million yearly saving, the Department expecting in fact a five-to-one ROI on the software within a six-year contract period. Some healthcare providers complain about the subjectivity of claims assessment in prepayment fraud-detection exercises, regarding for examples, excessive consultation, or patient over-treatment, and advice the software is better able to tell the difference between fraud and accidental billing mistakes. These are concerns which no doubt warrant looking into to make such software even more valuable while avoiding fortuitously labeling healthcare providers as fraudulent. Nonetheless, the role that such software could play in streamlining expenses in government initiatives as well, for examples, Medicaid and Medicare, which could make funding LTC easier is not in doubt. Governments in many developed countries are actually starting to acknowledge the important role healthcare ICT could play in addressing the multifaceted issues confronting contemporary healthcare delivery and investing substantially in these technologies. The U.K. government in 2002, for example, announced the biggest sustained spending growth in National Health Service (NHS) history, health spending up from 7.7% to 9.4% of gross domestic product (GDP) over 5 years, 2002-2003 to 2007-2008[13]. A major component of this spending rise was the recognition of the need for more ICT deployment in healthcare delivery the costs, a projected 4% increase of the entire budget, in a decade, an investment of about £18 billion (US $32 billion) for all NHS ICT spending, including on the national program. The goal of this national program is to link via a national information network, 36 000 GPs in over 8000 practices and 270 acute hospitals, community, and mental health facilities in the country[13]. Many other developed countries are starting to invest significantly in healthcare information and communication technologies, such investments no doubt likely to be of particular benefit in long-term care where a variety of different professionals are members of a multidisciplinary team often involved in the care of LTC patients. The need for effective information communication and sharing among such disparate groups, typically geographically dispersed, involved in the care of these patients, many with multiple chronic illnesses is not in doubt. Nor are the chances of reducing the often-significant transactional costs associated with care delivery in such circumstances. By helping to reduce morbidities among LTC patients for example, these technologies would be making it less expensive to provide care to long-term care patients, and with the quality of service provision actually enhanced, morbidity would decline even further, which would reduce health spending even further. This reduction in health spending would also reflect in a fall in the funds these patients, and their families and relatives spend on LTC, obtaining an even higher quality of care. This should reassure us about not panicking regarding the results of such as studies as one America's Health Insurance Plans (AHIP) released in October

2006, which found a provision in a health care information technology bill (HR 4157) passed earlier in 2006 by the House, could raise U.S. health care costs by as much as $416 million[14]. AHIP President and CEO Karen Ignagni wrote in an Oct. 12 2006 letter to lawmakers, that the study, which HayGroup prepared, found 'the near-simultaneous adoption of the new transaction standards and the new coding standards could potentially increase the cost for implementation by $115 million to $416 million.' The AHIP president noted that the October 2010 deadline for implementation of the new billing codes was not realistic, because it did not recognize the massive systems changes the clinicians, institutions, health insurance plans, vendors and other partners would need to implement before making the transition to the new codes. She recommended extending the deadline for implementing the new billing codes by another two years. Besides the argument for long-term benefits of initial investments, the question regarding what difference two years would make versus the four these organizations still have to make the systems changes and implement the appropriate healthcare ICT, would no doubt arise, again, initial investments that would no doubt pay off in the long term. These developments underscore the need for urgent measures to promote the widespread diffusion of these technologies in the health sector. Incidentally, the law, passed on July 27, 2006, would codify the Office of the National Coordinator for Health Information Technology within HHS, institute a committee to recommend on national standards for medical data storage, and establish a lasting structure to govern national interoperability standards, all key aspects of facilitating healthcare ICT use from which LTC would no doubt benefit. The law would also make clear that present medical privacy laws apply to electronic data storage and transmission, and obligate the HHS secretary to recommend to Congress a privacy standard to align federal and state legislation, also crucial to the widespread adoption and utilization of these technologies, including in the LTC domain. As the AHIP president noted, the number of billing codes providers employ to file insurance claims would increase due to the provision in the law on billing codes, the law also containing an exemption of anti-kickback laws that would enable hospitals to provide healthcare ICT hardware/software to doctors. Interestingly, another bill S 1418 the Senate passed in November 2005 did not have these two provisions, and efforts by the two law-making bodies to resolve the differences between the two laws are still afoot. The recognition of the importance of this reconciliation is evident in the letter to lawmakers written by a coalition of manufacturers and medical and business groups on October 11, 2006 requesting them to approve a final health care IT bill when they return on November 13, 2006 for a lame-duck session. The coalition that include the American Academy of Pediatrics, Dell, the National Association of Manufacturers and the U.S. Chamber of Commerce noted, 'seizing this important opportunity will move us one step closer to transforming a disconnected health system to one that promises substantial improvements in quality, safety and efficiency for America's patients and higher value for private and public payers.' There is no doubt that thus, that promoting the widespread diffusion of healthcare information and communication technologies is a significant approach to consider in our efforts to seek funding for LTC without compromising the quality of care delivery. This approach, exemplifies the need for the all-inclusive overall approach to this issue mentioned earlier, an important element of which is for us to first attempt to understand in detail the issues specific and general, to the long-term care constituent of a particular healthcare jurisdiction. Thus all concerned with LTC in that jurisdiction need to conduct a process cycle analysis of the particular sector of the LTC domain in which they are involved. This analysis, which essentially comprises identifying the main issues, decomposing them, thereby exposing the underlying issues and processes involved is important to reducing transaction-related costs. This is because such decomposition/exposition exercises would reveal the bottlenecks and problem areas in the entire transactional processes, thereby not only revealing that they need to address but also how, including the appropriate healthcare information and communication technologies that need implementing to achieve these goals.

N o doubt, there have been efforts at improving the quality of care delivery to

long-term care patients in many countries, for example in the U.S., those that laws such as the federal Nursing Home Reform Law effective October 1990, spawned, increased emphasis on patient evaluations and care planning, less use of physical restraints, and new standards of care, for examples. Seniors and others requiring LTC could also have more options, including receiving it a less institutional, assisted-living setting, or even at home. Some worry however, about the seeming efforts by both federal and state governments in the U.S, for example, in promoting certain of these options in response to concerns about finances and the imminent retirement of millions of baby-boomers, options they consider less expensive, exclusionary, and of defective quality[15]. The Medicaid Home and Community-Based Services (HCBS) waiver for example some argue is more flexible than Medicaid for example, honoring the rights of Medicaid recipients to receive essential nursing home services, simultaneously offering them a comparable care level at home or in an assisted-living facility, although some are wary of the commitment to quality standards with these waivers. Indeed, the Government Accountability Office in a 2003 report observed the lack of information on and oversight by the federal Medicaid program over care quality HCBS waiver funding provides. Such concerns make many question the wisdom in providing those in need of LTC vouchers to purchase needed services, and in the planned extensive supposedly flexible and easier to manage 'demonstration' waivers of federal Medicaid law by some states such as Florida, Kentucky and Idaho, implemented via Medicaid's demonstration waiver not HCBS waiver authority. These states would, under this statutory provision be able to ask the federal CMS for authority to initiate experimental programs not obliged to comply with Medicaid quality standards, and expunge recipients rights to some types of care, such as nursing home care, or raise cost sharing, even limit state or federal spending for recipients/services. These are reasons many object to the granting of requests by states for such waivers, which essentially could deny those in need of LTC, most of who cannot afford to pay for these services on their own, Medicaid coverage. Clearly, and as we noted earlier, pursuing options that would enable the achievement of the dual healthcare delivery objectives (DHDO) would serve not just the interests of these individuals and their families better but indeed those of society at large. Granting demonstration waivers for example that for Vermont recently which would offer all Medicaid LTC recipients a choice between HCBS waivers and nursing facility care while removing their rights to nursing facility services, except funds are available could essentially be counterproductive to achieving the DHDO in the long term. This is not mentioning the difficulties recipients that might need the excluded services would encounter. Besides exclusion, there are in fact also quality control issues regarding these waivers, in particular with budgetary constraint seemingly a key issue underlying the waivers, some concerned about mass movement to assisted-living facilities, most of questionable quality standards, with minimal if any nursing involvement or training for the staff there, for example, of Medicaid recipients from nursing homes. With monthly private-pay rates of nursing homes in the U.S., anywhere between 3 and over ten thousand dollars, the number of those requiring LTC that would not receive it due to these high costs in the country would run into millions, in particular with the imminent retirement of baby boomers. Further, LTC insurance, which as we also earlier noted covers only few persons, adverse selection issues driving up the costs of premiums relentlessly, and pay minimally on these services, roughly below 10% of LTC costs typically, and Medicare LTC coverage quite restricted. With even many hitherto financially sound seniors ending up on Medicaid, not least with the lists of medical conditions many have increasing with age, and correspondingly their healthcare bills and what Medicare could cover, that we need a radical re-conceptualization of LTC to avert an imminent crisis in the U.S., and indeed, many other developed countries is not in doubt. There is an urgent need for example, to address financing issues relating to LTC with a view to making services accessible on the one hand and to delivering these services in the most effective and efficient manner. There is little doubt if any that the widespread implementation of healthcare information and communication technologies would play a significant role in this regard. With research evidence indicating that these technologies could help in improve the efficiency and quality of care delivery, they could eventually help reduce healthcare costs, hence health spending as well. Thus, while helping to avert the financial problems the budgetary crunch mentioned earlier occasions, they do not compromise the quality of care, and indeed, improve it. There are of course several other approaches to addressing the key issues threatening to cripple long-term care in developed countries and different countries would have to seek the most suitable approaches in solving their specific problems. For example in some countries, obligatory and universal public social insurance programs pool the risk among all in society. Still in America, the Federal Accounting Standards Advisory Board (FASAB) recently recommended to Congress that deficit estimates include future Social Security and Medicare benefits-costs, and current benefits. This change in accounting practices would no doubt have significant implications for LTC funding in the country, not to mention its potential political fallout, which might determine at least in part, the acceptance or otherwise of the recommendations in the first place. With many other countries considering social insurance a political pledge to pay future benefits as opposed to being a financial liability, one cannot discountenance the role of political expediency in what some would consider an otherwise reasonable recommendation with the potential to strengthen accountability in the country's spending, including on LTC. This would necessitate cost-effectiveness in expenditures on services, hence the need to pay more attention to means by which we could achieve the DHDO, including investing in healthcare information and communication technologies. More broadly speaking, considering these benefits as liabilities creates an obligation government would not in future be readily able to slash, if it did not scrap Social security, and might therefore be more willing to tax. This is a dilemma that the achievement of the DHDO would be able to ease for example obviating the need to increase taxes, by reducing health spending, not compromising care delivery in the process. Furthermore, the health system makes intrinsic adjustments that make it less vulnerable to seeming pledges of future income that might not materialize with these benefits deemed liabilities. In other words, considering the multifarious factors that could potentially swing health spending back and forth, one would be hard-pressed to claim to be able to make accurate projections of its needs for funds. Yet, the health system should aim, and in part for these reasons, in case Congress accepts those recommendations, which it likely would, to achieve the dual healthcare delivery objectives on an enduring basis. This would make it less likely to need as much funds as the previous years assuming, albeit theoretically that it was able to continue to improve the quality of health services delivery, including in long-term care. This continuous improvement in service quality would translate in the long-term to improvement in the overall health of the populace, including that of seniors and the other categories of individuals that require long-term care. Improvement in health means fewer illnesses, hence less costs incurred, hence less spending on healthcare delivery. These issues underscore the point we made earlier about having a broader perspective on issues relating to long-term care, in particular considering the dynamics of health and healthcare delivery on the one hand and of both and progress in information and communication technologies on the other. We cannot ignore these important interrelationships in how we perceive and organize healthcare delivery at all levels in future, more so vis-à-vis the demographic changes many of the countries in the developed world are experiencing, not to mention the budgetary pressures under which they increasingly operate, the health and social benefits long enjoyed threatened by changes in the politico-economic domain. Furthermore, a healthier population would able to work longer, reducing the need for early retirement, and the likelihood of retirees requiring long-term care, or at least how much of it they would require, the realization of which is informing moves in countries such as Canada where Saskatchewan and other provinces are seriously considering increasing the retirement age. Another recent legislation in the U.S., the Deficit Reduction Act (DRA) of 2005, and turned law in February 2006, although disputed, also has significant implications for Medicaid long-term care policies, long-term care 36% of Medicaid expenditure spending, more than $100 billion yearly, which many of Medicaid's most expensive recipients, poor seniors and persons with disabilities use. Interestingly, the dispute has to do with the different forms in which the Senate and Congress passed the bill, differences that not only make some question its legality, but which the Congressional Budget Office (CBO) says would affect $2 billion in federal spending, issues regarding these differences probably going to require the intervention of the courts. Medicaid, which contributes significantly to LTC, which typically requires assistance provision regarding activities of daily living, for example, with dressing, bathing, bathroom use, meals preparation, medication use, home and money management, although not exclusive to these activities and managing money, would undergo major schisms under the DRA. These schisms, such as asset transfers, which among others extends the look-back period for asset transfer to assess Medicaid eligibility to five from three years, requires annuities disclosure and naming Medicaid a beneficiary for costs of Medicaid assistance, and excludes coverage for individuals with home equity over $500,000 or up to $750,000 at state option, are instructive. Essentially, the Congress has made significant alterations via DRA to the rules binding on states

32

regarding extending Medicaid eligibility. Other key areas are long-term care partnership programs, Family Opportunity Act, money follows the person demonstration, state options to provide HCBS services, and cash and counseling option. It has changed the dynamics between Medicaid and private long-term care insurance, and established new inducements and openings for states to veer Medicaid LTC services towards community-based from nursing-homes based. These all parts of efforts, which we noted before were inevitable, to limit federal and state financing commitment or at least, direct it to the most cost-effective and advantageous services for those needing LTC. In essence, the efforts aim to achieve what we termed the dual healthcare delivery objectives (DHDO), in which as we noted earlier the widespread implementation and use of healthcare information and communication technologies could play a significant role. This is even more so, with the shift in emphasis to the community with the likely increasing need for effective and timely communication between the many and disparate caregivers that would be involved in LTC provision in circumstance designed to limit access to institutional care, in effect to save money still delivering needed care.

The aforementioned underscores the point about the importance of revisiting

LTC funding and determining the appropriate approaches to this funding based on the realities of contemporary times. This is why some support the changes DRA occasions on Medicaid, for example, making it difficult for those who really do not need to be on Medicaid to be there by making eligibility standards tighter for individuals transferring assets. This is in contrast to present standards that allow well off individuals who could pay for their LTC, some divesting substantial amounts of money to be eligible for Medicaid, which critics consider these individuals know, would buffer their failure to plan appropriately for their future. Also unlike before when Medicaid did not consider the full value of any primary residence, persons with substantial home equity are ineligible for Medicaid LTC services, under the DRA it does, with an exception, a spouse or child with a disability lives in that home. Issues pertaining to long-term care, including funding issues are not peculiar to the U.S. Major Issues also confront facility-based long-term care in Canada for example, with variations in care delivery across jurisdictions, which the Canadian Healthcare Association (CHA), in its 2004 Policy Brief, *Stitching the Patchwork Quilt Together: Facility-Based Long-Term Care within Continuing Care - Realities and Recommendations*, described in depth. The CHA indeed, put forward a policy framework aimed at tackling these problems to enhance the flexibility of long-term care systems across Canada to enable them meet regional realities, while delivering equivalent services, proposals the National Advisory Council on Aging (NACA) fully backed[16]. Among the main defects in facility-based long-term care in Canada identified by the CHA, include the lack of public funding and affordability in institutional long-term care, rooted in the fact that facility-based long-term care is not a publicly insured service under the *Canada Health Act.*, hence is an assortment of services cross country, with different rates. Out-of-pocket costs average $18.00 per day in the Yukon (2004), and $137.00 per day in New Brunswick (2005), for examples[16]. The result though is the same for individuals that need these services, in particular, seniors, essentially limited if any access to qualitative, affordable and equitable facility-based long-term care, to address which provinces such as New Brunswick carries out an income and asset test to determine the resident's out-of-pocket expenses. However, this test, considered the most stringent in the country could end up stripping a resident's family of virtually all their assets to pay out-of-pocket expenses for a family member in an LTC facility. It is little wonder that the CHA proposed federal funding in keeping with the Canada Health Act for LTC institutions, and the funding of health services (personal care and health care services) in LTC facilities, which again highlights the issue of the need for aiming to achieve the dual healthcare delivery objectives, which would make such funding easier. In other words, the more money the health system is able to save while not diminishing the quality of health services it provides the people, including those in LTC facilities, the easier would be the funding of healthcare delivery in general, including LTC. This means that Canada should also start to explore ways by which it could achieve the DHDO, including for example, the implementation and utilization of healthcare information and communication technologies including in the delivery of long-term care services. Lack of quality care in institutions and accountability by care providers is another problem that CHA highlighted, and for which it proposed a range of measures to stipulate standards of care delivery, and quality assessment and control, including accreditation, training, and adequate staffing, among others, which again speaks to the need for achieving the DHDO. There is no doubt about the need of each jurisdiction to identify the key challenges confronting it in its efforts to deliver qualitative long-term care, and attempt to deal with the challenges as it best suits the particular jurisdiction. The country would also have to deal with the funding issues mentioned earlier and work with the private health insurance sector to streamline out-of-pockets costs across the country, while not compromising the standards of care delivered in long-term care facilities. The country is also going to face the challenges of large numbers of baby boomers retiring soon, and of more seniors that would require long-term care. It cannot afford to have these individuals not able to access the services that they need, hence would not to confront LTC delivery issues sooner than later. As noted earlier, there is much talk in the country, in particular in provinces such as Saskatchewan to increase the retirement age, hence give those seniors still fit and interested in holding on to their jobs or even seeking new ones to do so. This would encourage individuals to take health and wellness more seriously that intend to continue working past the current retirement age, and indeed, all persons, knowing that this could mean not needing LTC, or at least delaying when they would. Efforts invested in health promotion in this regard, including the deployment of any of the varieties of the increasingly sophisticated multimedia healthcare Information and communication technologies now available in achieving this goal, paying off, and indeed, helping to reduce health spending as healthcare costs falls, eventually. Thus, regardless of the funding system of a country's healthcare services, virtually all developed countries could expect a significant increase in the population of their seniors in the years ahead. These increases would have profound effects on their health systems, including on long-term care delivery. They ought to, therefore, be already exploring their options in tackling the imminent challenges this would spawn down the road. Addressing theses challenges successfully would warrant a major rethinking of long-term care services, at conceptual, strategic, tactical, operational, and at other levels. It would require both preventive and curative approaches taking into consideration the peculiarities of the particular health jurisdiction in question, for example, whether the health system's funding model is public, private, or mixed, and include other aspects of the administration of the health services, among others. Regardless of the context though, what each country wants to achieve is not having its retired seniors and others, including children that are sufficiently cognitively impaired or disabled in other ways as to require assistance not to have access to such services because they could not afford them. As noted earlier, it would be necessary to differentiate the levels of disability for example, and not just lump every one together and cart them to nursing homes, or move them out en masse of nursing homes into assisted-living facilities. By understanding each person's needs, it would the easier to optimize service provision, and develop these services to meet defined quality standards, and to provide each individual with the services needed efficiently and cost-effectively. It would be possible for example, to determine who would need to be in a nursing home, and who could receive services at home, under supervision, and what services each needs, and who should deliver them, and the level of training such providers need to have. This would also be beneficial to caregivers, as this would prevent the frustration and burnout that many experience providing care for which they have little or no training. Thus, we cannot afford to approach the problems of LTC delivery in isolation. We need to acknowledge the fact that these services would have to be multifaceted and linked someway in the future to make them more efficient and cost effective. We also need to recognize the pivotal role that a variety of healthcare information and communication technologies would play in this regard, for communication between disparate caregivers, for example, and for communication between patients and caregivers, for example, monitoring seniors' vital signs, even preventing and attending to falls. These are all efforts that would reduce the immense transactions costs involved in healthcare delivery in general, including long term care delivery that are soaring health spending currently and would likely worsen in the years ahead were we not to do anything to about it. It is important therefore to recognize the link between many of the issues confronting long-term care and the availability or otherwise of funding for these services, among others. Even attitudinal change among nurses and aid in nursing homes, which many have observed, requires measures in the educational domain, with implications for funding, in training these staff properly to meet the no-doubt potentially exhausting and yet rewarding enterprise of caring for seniors often with multiple health problems and other persons with disabilities requiring LTC. The issues are doubtless complex and require the concerted efforts of all stakeholders, in the health and indeed, other domains in the country, for example, the industrial and private sectors in general. This is why one of the first things we need to do is to educate the public on these issues and many of the measures each jurisdiction would take regarding solving this funding issue would likely affect everyone in the country. Here again, the role of healthcare ICT in the public awareness improvement drive is not in doubt. The point then is that as with the other aspects of healthcare delivery, these technologies have important roles to play in the future of long-term care delivery, and not only should developed countries in particular acknowledge this fact, but they should also act on it in devising solutions to an imminent long-term care crisis we should rather avert.

References

1. Iijima, Setsu. Future issues for the long-term care insurance system in Japan. Nippon Ronen Igakkai Zasshi - *Japanese Journal of Geriatrics*. 43(4):481-4, 2006 Jul.

2. Endo, Hidetoshi. Reconstruction of the long term care insurance system in Japan. Nippon Ronen Igakkai Zasshi - *Japanese Journal of Geriatrics*. 43(4):469-71, 2006 Jul.

3. Cramer AT. Jensen GA. Why don't people buy long-term-care insurance? *Journals of Gerontology* Series B-Psychological Sciences & Social Sciences. 61(4):S185-93, 2006 Jul.

4. Macdonald AJD, Carpenter GI, Box O, Roberts A, Sahu S. Dementia and use of psychotropic medication in non-'Elderly Mentally Infirm' nursing homes in south east England. *Age Ageing* 2002; 31: 58-64

5. Dyer. O. UK is urged to rethink funding of long term care of elderly people. *BMJ* 2006; 332:1052 (6 May), doi:10.1136/bmj.332.7549.1052-c

6. Available at: http://www.euractiv.com/en/socialeurope/eu-social-protection-expenditure-rise/article-159368?_print Accessed on November 5, 2006

7. Nuttall SR, Blackwood RJL, Bussell BMH, Cliff JP, Cornall MJ, Cowley A, et al. Financing long-term care in Great Britain. *Journal of the Institute of Actuaries* 1994; 121:1-53.

8. Available at:
http://www.oecd.org/searchResult/0,2665,en_2649_201185_1_1_1_1_1,00.html
Accessed on November 5, 2006

9. Shreeve M. An overview of provision for those in the 4th age. In: The 4th age in the 3rd millennium. Winchester: Brendoncare Foundation 1995: 10, 16.

10. Shaw AB. Age as a basis for healthcare rationing: support for agist policies. *Drugs Aging* 1996; 9: 403-405

11. Available at: http://www.cato.org/pub_display.php?pub_id=6728 Accessed on November 8, 2006

12. Available at:
http://www.usatoday.com/tech/news/computersecurity/2006-11-06-medicare-usat_x.htm?POE=TECISVA Accessed on November 9, 2006

13. Chantler, C., Clarke, T., Granger, R. Information Technology in the English National Health Service. *JAMA*. 2006; 296:2255-2258.

14. Available at:
http://www.kaisernetwork.org/daily_reports/rep_index.cfm?DR_ID=40745
Accessed on November 10, 2006

15. E.C. King, Rethinking Long-Term Care, The Commonwealth Fund, December 2005

16. Available at: http://www.naca.ca/expression/18-4/exp18-4_insert_e.htm Accessed on November 11, 2006

The New Healthcare Consumerism

The emerging consumer-directed health plan market in the U.S., now 6% of

all health plans in the country, and projected to grow to 25% by 2010 is not ignorable[1]. Governments, health plans, healthcare providers and consumers, employers, financial establishments, and other stakeholders would no doubt have to start paying attention to this phenomenon in the years ahead. With the need to provide qualitative health services, to rein in runaway health spending, to facilitate rational decision making by healthcare consumers on choice of providers for example, and in planning for healthcare costs, among main healthcare delivery concerns and increasingly so, developments in healthcare consumerism would have profound implications for the future of the health industry. The healthcare consumer's expectation of health services is increasingly sophisticated, and the need to make the right healthcare delivery choices more pressing. Today's healthcare consumer would progressively more be looking for the provision by relevant firms of a variety of services that would help in this regard, for examples, decision support technologies that assist in the choice of healthcare providers, fund tax-preferred accounts, prescription medications, health insurance coverage, medical/surgical services pricing, health content provision, and personal health records (PHR), among others. The use of consumerism here is in its economic sense, to emphasize the inevitable centrality of the healthcare consumer and of his or her ability to choose freely in the future of not just healthcare delivery, but also of the health industry and in the intricate interplay of this industry and other sectors of the economy. How for example, this centrality would be pivotal in the decisions of a healthcare organization on which software to purchase and whether to purchase it from a single vendor or from multiple vendors on a best-of-breed basis, based on its strategic healthcare delivery objectives, even on existential exigencies, its dwindling healthcare consumer patronage whose call for novel value propositions, starker. The implications of such decisions for competitiveness and product/service differentiation, and for prices falling, hence for the widespread diffusion of healthcare information and communications technologies (ICT,) would be likely remarkable. For example, would they not have implications for all healthcare stakeholders, including the healthcare consumer, who might then be able to establish connections with the technologies their healthcare providers have recently implemented, which would give them access to vital information about the providers crucial to decision making on choice for services for example? The increased placement of the healthcare consumer at the center of the healthcare-delivery enterprise therefore does not just have consequence for healthcare delivery, which incidentally it is shaping equally profoundly. It would in fact do so even more in future as the outcomes of the interchange of factors between the many industries involved in the varieties of transactional activities necessary and that culminate in healthcare delivery become manifest, for example, the relative buoyancy or otherwise that the competitiveness or lack of it in the automobile industry engenders. How would for example, the emerging healthcare consumerism influence our abilities to pay for health services for the millions of seniors that would retire in the next few years, for long-term care for example, for those of them that would need it? How could it help reduce health spending on the seniors and in fact, in general without compromising the quality of healthcare delivery? What potential influence could the freedom of the healthcare consumer to choose have on a country's competitiveness in the global markets? International trade in goods and services is a key element of the globalization process, to which that OECD countries' volume of world merchandise trade in the late 1990s was 16 times that in 1950, its credence in world GDP merely tripling in the same period, for example, attests[2]. In understanding the full ramifications of healthcare consumerism, we would need to have a broad concept of what constitutes this emerging phenomenon, including for example, conceptualizing healthcare consumerism as culture, part of emergent cultural milieu tied to a variety of other developments in society in eclectic domains, for example, the Web 2.0 phenomena. Would it be surprising therefore for us to find in the near future that social networking sites, tag-based folksonomies, bogs and wikis, and eventually fully operational semantic web technologies have become veritable sources of health information that play significant roles in the healthcare delivery choices of healthcare consumers? What implications would the potential healthcare consumer culture of the future have for the health industry, and indeed, for the entire economy? This 'culture' would no doubt be significant for the well-being of both the individual and society, hence not one we could discountenance. It could for example offer the health system, in a generic sense, a genuine opportunity to 'take' healthcare to segments of society contextually, based on their respective needs, making creating in the process, initiatives for example in healthy living and wellness possible that would otherwise be a chore. The potential for such initiatives for example to prevent diseases and improve health would indeed, be immense and their outcomes likely significant in achieving the dual healthcare delivery objectives (DHDO) of qualitative health services provision simultaneously reducing health spending, as the costs subsequent upon diseases declines with the corresponding fall in the disease prevalence. The loyalty to products and services in this context of consumerism would therefore be positive, even the risks of branding attenuated by the motivation for the loyalty, which even if it were rank enhancing, produced value for the money spent on it, for example, the qualitative services provided by one hospital, with post-surgery success rates healthcare consumers could confidently ballyhoo. The face of the new healthcare consumerism would therefore be in the main rooted in exigencies rather than frivolities, an attempt by the increasingly suave healthcare consumer to obtain best-of-breed services at bargain prices, the results of the ensuing transactions that would augur well for the entire health system, including other healthcare stakeholders and indeed, for the entire economy, eventually. No doubt, such 'informed' and 'voluntary' transactions benefit all concerned, as Adam Smith, the Scottish political economist (1723-1790) once noted. Furthermore, the exigencies mentioned earlier are common to both principal and agent in the transactions, hence the likely presence of stakes that would ensure the efficiency, hence cost-effectiveness of these transactions. The costs which as North (1990) [3] observed, guzzles a significant proportion of the gross national product (GNP) of many developed countries, could be substantial in healthcare delivery transactions. Thus, the underlying streaks of the efforts at rational decision making by the healthcare consumer that motivates the pursuit of excellence in healthcare delivery, which informs those by the healthcare provider to retain at least break-even patronage, purchasing particular healthcare ICT, are evident in those by the health system to achieve the DHDO. It is instructive therefore for promoting the pervasiveness of the centrality of the healthcare consumer that the health system transitions in a cascade of paradigms along a quality improvement continuum in tandem with technological progress, both driven by the increasing suaveness of the healthcare consumer manifested in the complexity of service expectations. It does not appear that there would be any stopping this transition, the evolving healthcare consumer expectation itself a product of the inter relationships of a variety of health and non-health factors, internal and external to the health industry, besides that of the symbiotic dyadic of the health system/healthcare delivery and technological innovation mentioned above. The imperative of quality then is harmonizing to the centrality of the healthcare consumer in the emerging healthcare delivery scheme. It is unlikely for example that many would contend the questionable sustainability of total health spending in the U.S., being 15.3% of the country's gross domestic product (GDP) in 2004, the highest percentage among Organization for Economic Cooperation and Development (OECD) countries, and over six percentage points more than the average of 8.9% in OECD countries[4]. Switzerland, Germany, and France spent 11.6%, 10.9%, and 10.5%, respectively. The U.S also spent over two times more than the OECD average in terms of total health spending per capita,US$6,100 adjusted for purchasing power parity, versus US$2,550 in the same year, and these figures continue to increase. Even considering that government revenues fund only 45% of health spending in the country, versus the OECD average of 73%, it is no doubt still substantial, versus the 37% funded by private insurance, still far more than in other OECD countries, even Canada, France, and the Netherlands, which with over 12% also have a fairly significant private health insurance involvement. Would it therefore be surprising to conceive of curtailing this spending, without compromising healthcare delivery, and in fact improving its quality by the state and federal governments in the country who are responsible for funding healthcare one way or another? Would it in fact not be even more expedient for these governments to act to overhaul the health system considering the limitation/lack of access to care by millions of its peoples despite these substantial investments in healthcare delivery, not to mention and as reasonable expectations would dictate considering the many not receiving adequate healthcare, health indicators that need improving? The initiation of efforts by the governments that would facilitate the achievement of the DHDO, which would somehow affect all the stakeholders involved, for example, promoting the widespread diffusion of healthcare ICT, would therefore be appropriate. With regards these technologies then, it would also be appropriate for the healthcare consumer to seek the best of the technologies required for the particular healthcare delivery related activity of interest. For example, the healthcare consumer that would acquire personal health records technologies, with which to connect not just to the healthcare providers' electronic health records (EMR), but also to the more national, as in the U.S., for example, National Health Information Network. Would it therefore not be necessary for the healthcare provider to do the same, regarding the EMR for example, as mentioned earlier, and would the healthcare providers in fact implementing and using technologies not predicate on the demands of their clientele, beside those of government initiatives aimed at achieving the strategic objectives of the health system? In other words, the impact of the new healthcare consumerism would traverse domains, motorizing the engine that would drive the changes that most health systems worldwide need to impel them into a future, the key aspect of survival in which would the capacity for flexibility and adaptability. The point here that healthcare delivery operating as a sacrosanct entity is moribund. The health system is going to have to acknowledge the new for appropriate policy changes in the new dispensation, in keeping with the rules of free market operations, which no doubt would not be a palatable proposition for many in the prevalent healthcare zeitgeist, but which nonetheless they prepare to accept, a conjecture reason would suggest.

The OECD and World Health Organization (WHO) in a recent report

commended the Swiss health system for meeting the significant objectives of good health outcomes and universal health coverage, but observed that the country's success was at a high financial cost, and recommended measures to control the country's high health expenditure[5]. The country has universal health-insurance coverage, its peoples could access a variety of modern health services, but spending an increasing proportion of its Gross Domestic Product (GDP) on health, the second highest (after the U.S. among OECD countries, many of which perform equally well, perhaps even better, at lower cost, speaks for itself. The country spent 11.5% of its GDP on health in 2003, versus the 8.8% OECD average, health spending, increasing by 2.4% of GDP from 1990 to 2004, versus the 1.5% OECD average, reflecting the bighearted supply and the high prices of services provision. According to John Martin, Director of the Employment, Labor and Social Affairs Directorate, OECD, regarding projected increase and the health system's financial sustainability, "Switzerland will have to develop more cost-effective policies if it wants to better control health expenditure in the future[5]". The report also noted that the country, despite high overall health spending, spends just 2.2% of this money on disease prevention and health promotion versus the 2.7% OECD average. Noted Dr. Marc Danzon, WHO's Regional Director for Europe, "Investing in prevention and health promotion programs would help Swiss health authorities focus on important public health issues such as tobacco and alcohol consumption and on areas in need of more attention such as mental health and obesity. This would promote health and prevent disease in the whole population, by actively targeting people at high risk." Many of the recommendations of the report attest to the point we made earlier about the increasing centrality of the healthcare consumer in the direction healthcare delivery would head in many countries, developed and developing, in the years ahead. It recommends the country adopting means to increase the cost-effectiveness of the Swiss healthcare system, for example. This no doubt would include measures to improve the efficiency of the variety of transactions conducted in the healthcare delivery process. Thus, it would warrant subjecting to scrutiny the elements of these transactions, including the authenticity, as flippant as it might sound, of the contact between the principal and the agent in these transactions, which for example, could influence adversely or otherwise the system of accountability in the entire system crucial for its survival. Thus the commitment or in fact its degree if at all, of the healthcare provider as an agent to the healthcare consumer or to the insurance firm or other healthcare purchaser would significantly influence the nature and quality of service delivery for example. These issues would influence in turn our approaches to policy changes in different domains for example that would move the respective domain closer to achieving its strategic objectives regarding the healthcare delivery enterprise. They bring to the fore the potential role of regulatory agencies, and who they are in the principal-agent interplay in reining in ex ante and ex-post transactional costs for example. The report mentioned above for example noted that present payment arrangements to both doctors and hospitals in Switzerland, namely fee-for service or by number of bed days, among others, lack the strong incentives to increase cost efficiency, hence the need for new methods of healthcare delivery payments, for example one based on fixed prices per pathology for inpatient care. The report noted that this would not only improve efficiency but also engender shorter hospital stays, as would greater use of gatekeeper or family doctors models and less fee-for-service payment models. Do these suggestions not confirm the need for the healthcare consumer to be central in the healthcare delivery scheme of things, if for example, the outcome of the commitment of the healthcare provider would be positive for the health system, which is crucial for it to be positive for its stakeholders? Would the payers not be paying more for health services for example, the healthcare consumer receiving sub-standard care, or not having the choice of provider or in matters relating to his or her health, with the likely increase in morbidities that would result? Would this consideration among others not have informed at least in part the recommendation in the report mentioned above regarding eschewing fee-for-service payment arrangements? Would a health system not be impelled to act regarding healthcare providers on whose watch health indicators are declining who nonetheless are receiving increasingly more payments, as some would insist, with the fee-for-service payment scheme, for example, say, practicing 'defensive medicine,'? Would there not be the need for implementing the appropriate healthcare ICT then that would facilitate evidence-based medical practice for example, or at the reimbursement end, those that would improve the efficiency of the claims processing, anti-fraud software and those patients could use to confirm procedures and services received? In other words, it would not in fact be in the interest also of the healthcare provider that the interests of the patient do not take center-stage in the healthcare delivery enterprise as not the provider's ethico-moral obligations, rooted in the Hippocratic Oath, mandate no wrongdoing to the healthcare consumer. Additionally, the worsening of the overall health of the people is a serious indictment of the failures inherent and imposed in the health system, to change which action becomes imperative, including strengthening the operations of the free market in the healthcare delivery domain, which would in any case place healthcare consumers where they belong, at the center of activities. Again, as the report noted, for the Swiss health system to curtail costs via competitive markets it is necessary to restrict the chances of insurers to selecting insurees based on their health risk, rather than contracting with providers based on quality, and that the healthcare consumer buying health insurance should shop for the best coverage at the least premium. It also recommended increased market competition for non-patented drugs, for examples, generics, which should slash medications prices. These recommendations emphasize a critical component of the centrality of the healthcare consumer in the healthcare delivery scheme, competition, which the new healthcare consumerism would necessarily spawn. By being able to choose healthcare providers, the healthcare consumer would be able to exercise discretionary powers that healthcare providers would ignore at their peril even in countries where public revenues fund the health system largely. Because health jurisdictions in these latter settings do have limited funds, and because many of them also have private health insurance and indeed, out-of-pocket funds involved in health services provision, they would over time even more acutely have to justify their very existence by providing services that their clientele needs, and that would keep them viable. Not so doing would no doubt diminish patronage. This would likely be so as options become available and affordable to the healthcare consumer, providers in the private sectors in these settings embracing the healthcare information and communication technologies for example that would enhance their service offerings in types and quality, prices falling with competition among them, their patronage increasing at the expense f the government hospitals. This scenario is already happening in some countries and health jurisdictions with hospital mergers and even closures, and would occur even more in the years ahead affecting health organizations that failed to become flexible and adapt to the changing times. This is likely to be even more so with the budgetary pressures that the projected increases in the population of seniors and the large numbers of retiring baby-boomers in the next few years would create. The key role of the healthcare consumer in driving competition among healthcare providers and payers, would be even accentuated in countries such as the U.S., where private funds constitute a significant percentage of health spending although, as noted above with health systems mostly funded by public funds, healthcare consumers would also play a major role among publicly funded health systems. Actualizing the mandates of the new healthcare consumerism would be therefore the responsibility of all the players in the healthcare delivery dynamics including the healthcare consumer.

Providing incentives for adherence to quality for example, is fine, but the quest for achieving the DHDO by the healthcare consumer is a strong reason to motivate the healthcare provider in a free market situation to improve value proposition and quality, to survive let alone thrive. Furthermore, imperfection is inherent in any health system, hence the need for enduring quality appraisal and improvement that constitute the foundation of the systems survival, too. Thus, for any health system to survive the changes internal and external to it, some anticipated others, catastrophic environmental accidents such as Hurricane Katrina or a Tsunami, hardly so, impose on it, there is no gainsaying the requirement for a continuous decomposition/exposition exercise that reveals its issues and processes and the changes they need to improve its quality. This process cycle analysis is therefore a crucial element in which every health system should engage tat would ensure the motivation for change not only remains strong, but also it drives and ensures that for quality improvement on a perpetual basis. No doubt, adequate reimbursement and incentives for excellent performance are important aspects of these quality improvement efforts, and require attention, as do other intermediate measures and processes relevant to ensuring the commitment of principals for example, to the contract with the agents. These measures are also potential drivers of the institution of the culture of duty, an extra effort in role performance that would accelerate the achievement of the DHDO in the long term. The healthcare provider by not embracing the healthcare information and communication technologies for example that could do the same would hinder its achievement, a scenario that although the emerging healthcare consumerism would increasingly make less prevalent compared to now.

The here is no doubt about the increasing recognition for example, of the benefits

of at least attenuating the problems relating to information asymmetry in the health industry, a relic of the paternalistic roots of the medical profession on the one hand, and of the disinterest in the healthcare ICT by many, capable of redressing these very problems. However, times are changing, and so are attitudes, not least due to efforts by various stakeholders to allay the fears of loss of privacy of personal health information for example, among the many concerns regarding these technologies. That local health information constitutes a major means of stressing current health issues and for health promotion and improvement, channel action for policy reappraisals, and enhance health initiatives in the community for example, is gaining currency. The example of an online, publicly accessible statewide portal offering zip code-level data, information, and maps for several health indicators attests to these changing times. The use of personal health records (PHRs), implemented in the Gulf region post-Katrina, WellPoint, one health plan actively involved, activating, its new PHRs, comprising claims data and member-provided information on roughly 18,000 employees of companies participating in a WellPoint pilot program, would likely become more widespread in time. Other instances point to the collaboration evident in many localities, and health jurisdictions that enhance the central place of the healthcare consumer in the healthcare delivery enterprise, for example the concerted efforts by a variety of healthcare stakeholders in Wythe County, to tackle the problems related to age-adjusted diabetes mortality rates in their community over twice that of the state[6]. Such efforts including screening for diabetes at health fairs by nurses, the hospital offering classes for persons recently diagnosed with the condition, the Chamber of Commerce, spearheading a social marketing effort plus worksite screening, health education on reducing its risks, and provision of prevention/treatment tools[6]. The role that healthcare ICT would play in this respect is self evident and no doubt significant, hence the need for continued efforts to promote the widespread adoption of these technologies, which would also help enhance the centrality of the new healthcare consumer in healthcare delivery. Also important in so doing is addressing the issue of expanding healthcare coverage to all Americans. With recent data from the U.S. Census Bureau indicating that, the number of persons lacking healthcare coverage increased by over a million persons in 2005 versus the previous year tackling this issue is indeed, urgent[7]. This is regardless of the fact that more persons obtained insurance coverage in 2005, 247.3 million, from just over 245 million in 2004, the percentage of uninsured increasing from 15.6% in 2003 to 2004 to 15.9%, presently, more so considering the economic growth and increasing employment during the year. The percentage of children without health insurance also increased in 2004/05, with 8.3 million persons below 18 years old lacking coverage in 2005, a manifestation of a lull in state initiatives on children's health insurance. Employer coverage has also been declining, down to 59.5% in 2005 from 59.8% the previous year, and that most of the uninsured affected employed adults suggests less employer-based insurance available, premiums, and copays increasingly not affordable. The high deductible health plans (HDHP), and health savings accounts characteristic of consumer-directed healthcare should avert these problems with time, although it seems rates increases, more stringent underwriting criteria, and certain states' coverage rules, among others, are coming in the way for now. This paradox in the latter is evident considering the need for states to achieve the DHDO, and the potential of this healthcare delivery model to contribute significantly in the achievement of these goals. The same holds for employers, the larger of which though continue to offer health coverage in the main, albeit still struggling with solutions to crippling health and retirement benefits in some cases, the problem mainly regarding the small and medium-sized enterprises (SMEs), which incidentally, constitute the bulk of the service industry in the country, as indeed, in other developed countries. In other words, our efforts need focused in particular on how to promote employer-based health insurance coverage among these employers, mostly entrepreneurs, the coverage for themselves and their families, besides their employees, the number of uninsured working-age Americans projected to be over 27miliion persons in 2006. The need for concerted efforts in this regard could not be clearer, discount coverage with chamber of commerce membership, helpful, at least until premium increases accentuates moral hazard those preferring private insurance leaving behind, typically older more ill members hardly able to afford the ever-increasing premiums. This underscores the need for federal legislative support for small business health plans (SBHPs) that would enable small-business owners to join forces across state lines to buy health insurance as a group. In the Senate's first floor action on SBHP in May 2006, it held a key vote on S. 1955, 'The Health Insurance Marketplace Modernization and Affordability Act of 2006,' the 55-vote majority acquired insufficient (60 votes required) to carry on under Senate rules[8]. As noted earlier, the link between healthcare delivery and the new consumerism is anything but tenuous. Developments in the clinical and other domains of healthcare delivery including for example in the economic, both domestic and in the broader global milieu puts the onus on us not only in the U.S., but in other countries as well, developed and developing, to ensure the delivery of qualitative health services and efficiently and cost-effectively too. The alternative would be nothing other than a descent into chaos not just in the health domain, the aftershocks of which in themselves are enough to rock some of the most cherished foundations of society, for example, the health, and wellness of its peoples, but also in other societal endeavors such as its economic growth and its sustainability. The mandate of the new healthcare consumerism stems therefore from our obligation to ourselves as humans, also though recognizing the interwoven nature of our individual interests with those of our fellow humans. It is therefore not solely to protect ourselves that we should acknowledge this emerging healthcare consumerism, but also in the acceptance of the new realities that confront us, how for example, someone contracting an unknown virus in a village in the Andes could be the start of a pandemic, in a world linked by jets by just hours. How different countries approach the issue of the centrality of the healthcare consumer in the new healthcare scheme would depend on a variety of factors, which as we have noted include health and non-health factors, internal and external to the particular health system or jurisdiction. In Canada, for example, where most of the funds for healthcare derive from public coffers, the principles entrenched in the Canada Health Act underline this centrality. It does not matter therefore that the provinces and territories directly administer health services these services must reflect the centrality of the healthcare consumer. The issue of healthcare consumerism however, is a different matter relative to countries such as the U.S., where private funding for healthcare are more prominent. Nonetheless, healthcare consumerism is emergent even in Canada, and would likely be even more so in the years ahead, with the increasing interest across the country in the private healthcare running in parallel with the public health system, or Medicare, as in Australia and New Zealand. The landmark Supreme Court decision in the Chaoulli v. Quebec case in June 2005, that Quebec should allow private health insurers to compete with the public system, in fact again brought the matter forward into public glare. The effect of this ruling is magnetic cross-country, Alberta coming up with its "Third Way" healthcare model, British Columbia's interest in private health delivery increasingly evident, even private firms springing up across the country venturing into the healthcare delivery business. Furthermore, most Canadians support the establishment of a parallel private health system in the country, according a 2005 Canadian Medical Association poll, 52% to be precise, although 54% consider it would compromise the public health system[9]. As previously noted, Medicare places the patient at the centre of healthcare delivery in the country, whose importance, to which the ruling, which it underpinned attests. With Quebecois now able, to pay for healthcare services covered by Medicare via private insurance, there is no doubt that the centrality of the healthcare consumer would be highlighted in this province, with potential consequences for improvement in the quality of care delivery and overall reduction in health spending by the province. The Quebec healthcare consumer would therefore now be able to choose between queuing on a long waitlist, that Mr. Zeliotis had to wait for over a year on such a list for hip surgery what triggered the lawsuit mentioned above in the first place, or opting to receive treatment outside the public health system using private insurance. In other words, market forces would become operational in Quebec, healthcare consumerism, bloom. Their ability to choose would mean that healthcare providers would have to convince healthcare consumers that they are the right choices. This would mean providing satisfactory services and beyond, for example, differentiating their services from those of their competitors via value propositions in which the implementation of sophisticated healthcare information and communication technologies would likely play a significant role, and justifiably so. Indeed, a recent study showed that even 'googling' and the use of web based searching could assist doctors to diagnose complex cases[10]. With internet access increasingly ubiquitous in outpatient clinics and hospital wards, would the World Wide Web not ever more serve important purposes in the clinical domain, and would the GP for example able to take this essentially most basic opportunity not have an edge over competitors struggling with diagnosis, ordering unnecessary lab tests, incurring avoidable costs? Is it not evident how the use of such basic and readily available healthcare ICT could help achieve the DHDO? Developments in non-health domains in the country, such as those announced on November 09, 2006, in the tax arena in Saskatchewan by Finance Minister Andrew Thomson, which would see the province's residents save \$28.1 million in personal income tax in 2007, as the provincial government indexes the Personal Income Tax (PIT) system to the national rate of inflation, are crucial. This is so as they would help keep workers and pensioners' buying power intact. The province plans to increase income tax brackets and tax credits for 2007 by 2.2%. The full indexation announced would also shield residents from 'bracket creep' wherein income tax credits fall and income taxes rise due to inflation-based adjustments to personal income[10] . This would hence avert the erosion by inflation of the value of income tax brackets, basic and spousal credits, senior supplement, dependent child credit, age credit, disability-related credits, medical expense credit and the provincial sales tax credit. There is no doubt that these tax cuts, over half-a-billion dollars in the past year alone, including cuts in property taxes, corporate taxes, small business taxes, sales taxes and this time income taxes, would stimulate economic activities in the province, including in the health industry. It would therefore be easier for residents to enroll with private health insurers for coverage of health services that Medicare does not cover, and because the funds are out-of-pocket and for which competing interests vie, we would again witness the operation of market forces. Thus, the healthcare consumer would likely seek real value for their money, healthcare consumerism, yet at play, the potential outcome for the private/public healthcare delivery dyadic likely to be a crucial contributor to the direction of healthcare delivery not just in the province, but cumulatively in the country in the coming years.

To underscore the important role that healthcare consumerism would play in the future of healthcare delivery, a recent report by First Consulting Group, *Consumer Driven Healthcare: It's Impact on Physicians,* noted that consumer-driven health (CDH)plans are, and would gain increasing currency in the business community[12] With CDH enrollment twice more than in the previous year, and total membership now between 5 million and 6 million, the plans estimated to constitute 12% of the private health insurance market by 2008, the increasing significance of the centrality of the healthcare consumer in the healthcare delivery scheme is indeed, evident. The report additionally, observed that focused healthcare ICT could assist doctors' practices tackle the pecuniary and management challenges CDH claims might pose, among others, which again highlights the need for recognizing the multifaceted impact of the rising healthcare consumerism, as noted earlier. The important roles that healthcare ICT would play in the many transactions, health and non-health speaks to why we should support efforts to promote the widespread diffusion of these technologies. As DeLeys Brandman, vice president for strategic sourcing and delivery at FCG Health Plans noted, "The arrival of consumer-driven health plans means that consumers will have more direct purchasing power in healthcare and they'll be looking to make sure they get appropriate value for their money." She added, "Providers need to come up with strategies to ensure they can deal with the changes." The point in fact is that this increasing centrality of the healthcare consumer goes hand in hand with a corresponding increase in the implementation and use of healthcare information and communication technologies. As the report also noted for example, a necessary aspect of the evolution of CDH is electronic information storage and exchange because of the likely need of enrollees in CDH plans to seek and expect to access quality and pricing information essential to a rational comparison of physicians and their services, hence to make the right choice of service provider. The report also recommended that physicians purchase electronic medical records, preferably an ambulatory system with e-prescribing and decision support features, and one able to document performance as an aspect of the overall care documentation process that would facilitate claims management. It also suggested the need for systems able to communicate with and share patient information with other providers, in other words able to integrate with for example, a statewide EHR system. These recommendations no doubt support our assertion of the potential for healthcare consumerism to drive progress in healthcare delivery, which in turn would stimulate innovation in healthcare information and communication technologies, for example, to address the challenges posed by revelations of the ongoing continuous quality appraisal efforts. The novel technologies that emerge would in turn spawn new ideas and approaches to care delivery and the process continues ad infinitum. Additional benefits, besides the improvement in the quality of healthcare delivery that would result from this process is the potential for prices of services to fall, as for example some doctors that now charge lesser fees to promote online consultation, with payers also starting to pay for e-consultations, all parties benefiting from the cost-savings. Thus, all parties would be contributing to one another's achievement of the dual healthcare delivery objectives. The concept of healthcare consumerism is thus clearly one that we should all promote and not eschew as its underlying principles and manifest benefits are in the best interests of the healthcare delivery efforts few if any would not consider worthwhile regardless of country or health jurisdiction. The results of a recent national survey on Americans' attitudes toward the financing and provision of health insurance is instructive on some of the salient issues tied to the emerging consumerism[13]. The survey conducted by researchers from University of Chicago's NORC, released on November 14, 2006 at a *Health Affairs* briefing in Washington D.C., and published as a November 14 *Health Affairs* Web Exclusive, showed that while healthcare consumers want more health insurance coverage and choice, they are not keen to pay more for health insurance. The survey also showed that the uninsured are likelier to reject policies that mandate the purchase of health insurance, and over 25% of Americans do not object to charging obese people higher premiums. Not only is the freedom to choose, the cornerstone of healthcare consumerism implicit in these findings, so is the need for achieving the dual healthcare delivery objectives. The desire of the American public for more coverage and choice is consistent with the elements of healthcare consumerism achievable via means by which the ability to choose providers for example places the healthcare consumer at the center of the healthcare delivery enterprise. Such means would be those that strengthen the operations of market forces, for example, that mitigates moral hazard, which the American public apparently implicitly supports according to the results of the survey regarding the obese. Such riders to health insurance and incentives for exercising regularly or for not smoking for examples, incorporated in health insurance contracts, would in turn mitigate adverse selection, and eventually drive down health insurance costs. The law of demand would kick in up to point, in the direction that might seemingly drive overall healthcare costs up on cursory examination, due to the fall in prices, but the change in the nature and extent of service utilization would mean that even the increased demand would ultimately drive down overall health spending as healthcare costs fall. Put differently, the healthcare consumer would be using health services more, but using different services, this time preventive and wellness services rather than the more expensive curative services due to the decline in diseases prevalence that the initial increased service use and more attention paid to disease prevention would engender. Furthermore, the increased availability of resources for other social and other services that would result from the decrease in overall spending would also boost health and wellness among the populace, resulting in a more productive, more economically buoyant society. This is why we cannot afford to ignore the health of essentially everyone in society, and we need to develop appropriate programs for facilitating access to care, as even those currently making little if any contribution to the economic progress of society could then be able to do so if healthy and strong. It is also, why, considering the importance of immigration to the economy of many countries, its effects, including those of illegal immigration on the society's overall health status, should feature prominently on the healthcare agenda. This is more so as these persons are integral parts of the emerging healthcare consumerism that we have been discussing. In the U.S., for example, it cost taxpayers $1.1 billion in 2000, according to recent Rand study published in the November/December 2006 edition of the journal Health Affairs, to fund healthcare for illegal immigrants[14], between 18 and 64 years old, or roughly $11 per household. The study noted that the cost in Los Angeles County in the same year was $204 million. However, the Federation for American Immigration Reform queried the study's findings, suggesting that these costs were miniscule, relative to how much the country spends on other social services for example, estimates for the total cost of healthcare for illegal immigrants in California alone, the Federation put at $1.4 billion. Costs apart, disputes over its exact amount regardless, as the Federation's Jack Martin observed, 'From the studies that we have done, (the Rand study) certainly is a low-ball estimate..., but there are issues other than cost.... In the emergency rooms, it has to do with very finite resources and the fact that those medical facilities end up at times being severely overburdened so that the quality of attention that they can give to U.S. citizens and legal permanent residents is degraded.' This is why this matter concerns the ramifications of healthcare consumerism in the first place, an essential aspect of which is a realistic approach to healthcare issues. The point here is that ignoring the healthcare needs of these individuals could only worsen the overall health of the American society as a whole. On the on the other hand, considering their health issues of warranting attention, would bring us closer to appreciating the full extent that healthcare consumerism could influence for the better, not just the country's health system, but its entire economy. The question therefore is whether we should worry about the costs of healthcare delivery to these persons or not, but rather how we could integrate health services provision to them into the overall healthcare delivery scheme. The Rand study surveyed Los Angeles County residents about their use of healthcare services and estimated the costs of care using national estimates on cost. It found that almost 22% of illegal immigrants have health insurance, costs, roughly $362 million in 2000, of which immigrants funded $321 million out of pocket. Would it not be preferable for all these immigrants to have health insurance, and would the funds infused into the system thereof not offset those of caring for a small minority of undocumented or poor immigrants, we could assume and safely so would still exist even then? Indeed, California's Medi-Cal program in 2004/05 paid $946 million in services for poor illegal immigrants. These funds covered services such as ER treatment, prenatal care, partial cancer treatment, abortions and nursing home care, Los Angeles County in 2003, $340 million for public hospital and clinic care for those of these persons lacking Medi-Cal bills for children and seniors included, but not in the Rand study. Furthermore, the number of illegal immigrants, and healthcare costs have soared in the five years since collecting the Rand data in 2000, whereas healthcare consumerism would do the reverse regarding costs, if we allowed the operations of market forces among these individuals. Consider for example, the finding of the Rand study that illegal immigrants consulted doctors less often than citizens did, which it explained as due to their younger ages, and the tendency for the frail and the elderly to stay back in their home countries, although it could be because these immigrants were trying to avoid arrest. Whatever the reason were however, there is no doubt that the more opportunities immigrants have to access healthcare delivery, the less it would cost both themselves and eventually the entire health system. Thus, it would be necessary to eschew role diffusion when it comes to health service provision for illegal immigrants, doctors, nurses, and other healthcare providers simply play their specific roles in health service provision, and doubling as cops or immigration officers. The argument here predicates on the benefits of the new healthcare consumerism, in other words, that the concept applies to all residents of any country, legal or illegal, as the majority of these persons contribute one way or another to the overall economic activities of the country.

The idea is not to condone illegal immigration, but to address the problems

associated with it in situ pending whatever solution to the issue of illegal immigration eventually emerges. Thus, as long as people live and work within the confines of a geographical territory, they are integral components of its organic structure. Every country should encourage such individuals to buy insurance coverage, and since most illegal immigrants are employees, albeit illegally, they earn money and should be able to purchase health coverage suited to their wallets. As noted earlier, the funds this affords the health system, in addition to the taxes that they pay, would significantly at least in the long term, take care of the health bills of those of them unable to purchase health insurance for a variety of reasons such as disability, or poverty. This is so because wit the operations of market forces as noted earlier, healthcare consumerism would eventually eliminate moral hazard, hence adverse selection, among the immigrant populations, and the healthier they become, the more would have jobs, the less would be ill health, and its associated costs, and hence the less the spending on healthcare for the poor immigrants. Clearly much work needs done beyond these high-level considerations, clearly best left to individual states to handle, with general guidelines for example on the parameters for encouraging immigrants to purchase health insurance coverage, vis-à-vis tax issues, funds repatriation, and other pertinent issues. All of these issues, once spelt out could in fact inherently control the flow of immigrants into and out of the country, of course with whatever policies instituted given legal teeth and enforced. It might be necessary for example to make it easier if not mandatory for illegal immigrants to work once they have insurance coverage, and for a specified period of time, depending on the nature of the coverage they acquired relative to their earnings, or to even regularize their stay on account of these and other relevant issues. The idea here is to acknowledge the difficult countries such as the U.S and Canada, for example, face with their extensive and porous borders regarding the issue of immigration, within the context of the exceedingly mobile labor force in our contemporary times, which is the first step toward addressing the issues in the most appropriate manner. While these countries would still have to police their borders, as allowing immigrants en masse in could overwhelm the health and social services, which unmistakably would be a recipe for chaos and potentially, societal disintegration. They would therefore need to find the most expedient formula to deal with the issue and since the burden of immigration on health services is a crucial aspect of the problems these persons might pose to any country, to consider some of the issues raised here regarding healthcare consumerism, as apposite. The essential background to this is the potential for healthcare consumerism, not just to ensure the achievement of the DHDO objectives by these and other countries dealing with such issues, but also in fact, that of the benefits of the economic productivity consequent upon their presence in the country. Both of these advantages, the issues, and processes involved with them if explored and implemented appropriately, including for example, regarding healthcare delivery, the contributions of healthcare information and communication technologies, would no doubt be critical aspects of a country's ongoing evolution toward sustainable economic growth and development. The recent approval by European health ministers from 53 countries of the world's first charter to fight obesity on November 16, 2006, attests to the significance of the 'inclusion' policy enunciated above regarding illegal immigrants. Drafted by the World Health Organization (WHO) in consultation with European countries, the charter, approved in Istanbul, Turkey, is the first genuine attempt to oblige national authorities to take tangible action to fight obesity. Observed Dr. Francesco Branca, the organization's European adviser for nutrition and food security, 'Lots of governments have good recommendations and nice guidelines, but in terms of nutritional goals, most countries haven't achieved them.' The charter obligates governments to take such measures as making healthy foods more available and regulations for safer roads to encourage more people to walk and cycle. These measures would no doubt 'include' and not exclude persons with overweight/obesity problems from the health system, but in doing so, discourage adverse selection, making health insurance more accessible to these persons and many others who would otherwise have not been able to afford one were the policy that of exclusion rather than inclusion. The prevalence of obesity in Europe is now thrice what it was twenty years ago, 50% of all adults, and 20% of children, overweigh, with implications for increased risk of developing chronic diseases for example, diabetes, heart diseases, and cancer, higher burden of diseases, in both psychological and pecuniary terms, and indeed, of mortality, oftentimes, prematurely. Indeed, obesity guzzles up to 6% of all health care costs in Europe, an 'epidemic' the Who charter hopes to contain in five years, although it might take no longer in more countries than in others, considering the logistics issues involved in the multi-sectoral efforts that implementing the charter would involve. It would indeed, require massive efforts including investing upfront as we noted earlier in relevant programs and technologies, such as healthcare information and communications technologies, critical to the 'mindset-changing' efforts. In other words, it would not be easy to reorient persons in a milieu where fast food chains are opening up outlets in virtually every street corner, fewer persons are exercising habitually, and more are embracing increasingly sedentary lifestyles. Nonetheless, the efforts would be worthwhile in the long term, with these patterns reversed and people live healthier. It is also important to focus on children among whom overweight/obesity is becoming increasingly major health issues. This not only results in the earlier onset of these chronic diseases, which with obesity likely remain with them into adulthood, issues that the charter, which also advocates precise regulatory measures directed at the private sector to 'substantially reduce' the advertising of unhealthy foods to children, aim to rectify. No doubt, such measures would antagonize the food industry, which perhaps explains the differences in approach to the issues in different countries with for example, Norway and Sweden banning advertising to children, versus in the Netherlands, Portugal, and Spain, for examples, where the food and drink industries self-regulate the industries. Considering the seriousness of what are at stake in health, economic and developmental terms, many feel strongly about the issue of advertising unhealthy foods and beverages to children, calling for such laws as the charter suggests. However, others feel that a more effective approach would be addressing the problems from the demand side, in other words, reducing the demand for such foods and beverages, which again, promoting healthcare consumerism would help achieve. Thus, would the health system, and of course, organizations and other stakeholders with the resources so to do, investing upfront in for example targeted and contextualized health information dissemination, regarding these unhealthy foods and beverages, not help reduce the demand for them, in particular? Would this not in fact even be likelier, coupled with the fact that the health insurance premium their families would pay would be increasingly less? Would parents not more likely join in the efforts to discourage on their children the effects of these advertising? In other words, with market forces operational, would healthcare consumerism not prevail, with children and their families, making more-rational choices regarding their health? Would the healthcare provider not likely introduce not just health education and promotion programs in the entire value proposition offered healthcare consumers, in particular, with such initiatives tied to performance evaluation and recompense? In short, any serious effort to address these problems, which many countries not just in the developed but also in developing countries face, would require promoting healthcare consumerism, via the operations of market forces. With their health and those of families members increasingly important and the potential for improving it increasingly clearer, the healthcare consumer would be more discerning not just in the choice of healthcare providers, but also in life's choices in general. Not that healthcare consumerism is some sort of 'silver bullet,' but as with the issues on immigration that we discussed earlier, promoting it would make addressing the health problems of the financially challenged in society much less difficult. In Europe, the estimated numbers of persons expected to be obese by 2010 are 150 million adults and 15 million children. Again, as Branca noted, 'Everyone says it takes a generation to reverse this, but it doesn't…..If we work together now, we might be able to change the obesity trend at the same speed at which it happened,' the massive increase in obesity occurring essentially just in the past ten years. Thus, there is a need to mobilize resources and efforts in addressing these and other health issues to prevent them becoming even more difficult to solve. The merging healthcare consumerism would play a key role in speeding up the reversal of trends that are unhealthy and could potentially create enormous disease burden. With the increasing spending on health in many countries, in particular in developed countries, with also the likelihood of health spending increasing even further in the years ahead with the increase in the population of the elderly, there is no doubt about the need to promote healthcare consumerism, and indeed, about doing so being imperative. This latter, is so as the world becomes increasingly competitive, and globalized. No country could afford not to be competitive in such a milieu, and to keep spending an increasing portion of its wealth, literally, on an increasingly unhealthy populace. Any country that does that would soon essentially consume itself in a vicious cycle of ill health and soaring healthcare costs, hence spending, simultaneously becoming less productive, hence less competitive, the resources to spend on health increasingly depleted, its populace even unhealthier. Would such a country not benefit from promoting healthcare consumerism, for example, its peoples equipped with the means, data and information, required to make rational choices regarding their health and who provides them healthcare? The point is that changes in the wider world are going to continue to impinge on all aspects of our lives in our domains. We would have little or no choice but to be cognizant of these changes and to incorporate in our lives those that would make us better adapted to survive in this wider increasingly transient world. This point underscores the efforts of organizations such as the Partnership for Clear Health Communication (www.p4chc.org), a national, nonprofit coalition of organizations whose aim is to build awareness and advance solutions to improve health literacy and to influence health outcomes in a positive manner. The strongest predictor of someone's health status is literacy skills, in particular, health literacy skills, in other words, the ability of the individual to read, understand and to take action on health data and information[16]. A 2003 National Assessment of Adult Literacy noted the literacy skills of 30 million Americans to be 'below basic,' persons so defined having problems understanding instructions for taking medications or even an appointment slip to see the doctor. The study also showed that 63 million Americans have 'basic level' literary skills, with problems calculating a dose of an over-the-counter medication for a child or understanding what a consent form is. These issues do not just affect the elderly and the poor, who tend to be overrepresented in such populations, and who incidentally are some of the heaviest users of health services, but cuts across ages, income brackets, and nationalities. Indeed, about half of those in the below basic and basic literacy levels are native-born, white adults. No doubt, other countries need to examine literacy issues as they constitute the most fundamental element of the emerging healthcare consumerism, and enable individuals to make the appropriate choices crucial to the evolution of the concept and all the benefits that could accrue thereof that we mentioned earlier. The Partnership for Clear Health Communication has developed a tool, Ask Me 3, which encourages patients to ask 3 questions at every healthcare visit: What is my main problem? What do I need to do? Why is it important for me to do this? The organization aims to improve the healthcare consumer's understanding of the healthcare process, hence empower the consumer to make the right choices, including asking additional questions, and seeking solutions to other health problems, both of the consumer and their families and others.

The significance of the need for health literacy might become clearer with the

example of say consumer X, who is an American male and has a primary and secondary insurance, but still ended up paying over half of the bills for a procedure, which turned out the consumer did not in fact need costing almost $10,000. Could this consumer, who had to borrow the balance from a friend, have paid less understanding the procedure was unnecessary and that there were less costly and equally reliable alternatives, even regarding insurance, taking up catastrophic coverage for example, rather than the primary and secondary insurance coverage? Does this example not highlight the need to promote healthcare consumerism, which would help solve both the problems of un-, and under-insurance and enable the achievement of the dual healthcare delivery objectives, at both the personal, health system, and other levels? Without access to healthcare by its peoples, no health system could claim to be a success, and could in fact avoid the ultimate degeneration described above into a vicious cycle with potential major adverse consequences not just for the health system, but also for the entire economy. One of the major obstacles of health system access as the case of consumer X above who seems not just to have the wrong insurance policies, but also who the health system seems to exploit shows, is the pervasive information asymmetry in health systems with roots in the paternalism inherent in the doctor-patient dyadic. It is therefore important in promoting healthcare consumerism to focus on rectifying this information asymmetry, which again as the example above shows, could result in the healthcare consumer paying more, and not health for services, and indeed, paying for services that they do not need, both counter to the tenets of healthcare consumerism, hence obstacles to enjoying its benefits. Thus, the important link between healthcare consumerism and the promotion of and widespread implementation and utilization of healthcare information and communication technologies in our contemporary times becomes evident. In other words, our efforts to improve health literacy would increasingly hinge on these technologies in an age when the technologies increasingly feature in every other aspect of our lives, and even more crucially, their use in achieving this goal, that of rectifying information asymmetry is likely to be more cost-effective and efficient. Would it not be more so for example initiating information dissemination electronically than via snail mail, not to mention the varieties of sophisticated multimedia portals via which we could achieve the same goal? This then is why and as a part of our efforts to achieve the dual healthcare delivery objectives (DHDO) it is important to acknowledge the role that these technologies would play and to promote their widespread diffusion among all healthcare stakeholders. They are the starting point in our quest to make healthcare consumerism more prevalent, to benefit from its positive influence on not just individual but societal health. The more we appreciate these important connections, and take the necessary measures toward making them work in tandem even more effectively, the closer we would be to achieving the dual healthcare delivery objectives that would be crucial to the survival of health systems worldwide in the years ahead.

References

1. Available at: http://www.healthcareitnews.com/story.cms?id=5853 Accessed
on November 11, 2006

2. Available at:
http://www.oecd.org/findDocument/0,2350,en_2649_34257_1_119693_1_1_1,00
.html Accessed on November 11, 2006

3. North, D.C., (1990). Institutions, Institutional Change, and Economic
Performance. Cambridge University Press, Cambridge.

4. Available at:
http://pdftohtml.markoer.org/pdf2html.php?url=http://www.oecd.org/datao
ecd/29/52/36960035.pdf Accessed on November 12, 2006

5. Available at:
http://www.oecd.org/document/47/0,2340,en_2649_201185_37562223_1_1_1_1,
00.html Accessed on November 12, 2006.

6. Luck, J., Chang, C., Brown, E.R., Lumpkin, J. Using Local Health Information
To Promote Public Health. Health Affairs; Jul/Aug2006, Vol. 25 Issue 4, p979-
991, 13p

7. Available at:
http://web.ebscohost.com/ehost/pdf?vid=30&hid=109&sid=63b2e270-b22d-
476f-bd2b-c216cdcc1d8a%40sessionmgr102 Accessed on November 12, 2006

8. Available at: http://www.ahpsnow.com/page/sbhpsnowCurrentStatus
Accessed on November 12, 2006

9. Available at: http://www.csmonitor.com/2005/0808/p06s01-woam.html
Accessed on November 13, 2006

10. Tang H, Ng JHK. Googling for a diagnosis - use of google as a diagnostic aid: internet based study. Br Med J doi:10.1136/bmj.39003.640567.AE (published 10 November 2006) Available at: http://www.bmj.com/cgi/eletters/bmj.39003.640567.AEv1#148937 Accessed on November 13, 2006

11. Available at: http://www.gov.sk.ca/newsrel/releases/2006/11/09-803.html accessed on November 13, 2006

12. Available at: http://www.healthcareitnews.com/story.cms?id=5907
Accessed on November 13, 2006

13. Berk, M.L., Gaylin, D.S., and Claudia L. Schur. Exploring The Public's Views On The Health Care System: A National Survey On The Issues And Options *Health Affairs*, 25, no. 6 (2006): w596-w606

14. Available at: http://www.latimes.com/news/health/la-me-health15nov15,1,1376312.story Accessed on November 16, 2006

15. Available at: http://news.yahoo.com/s/ap/20061116/ap_on_he_me/anti_obesity_charter&printer=1 Accessed on November 18, 2006

16. Rudd R, Kirsch I, Yamamoto K. *Literacy and Health in America*. Princeton:
Educational Testing Service; 2004.
Available at: http://www.ets.org/Media/Research/pdf/PICHEATH.pdf
Accessed November 18, 2006.

The Changing Face
Of
Health Economics

At the core of economics is the concept of scarcity, the lack of sufficient resources to satisfy all fully. No matter how rich or poor a country is therefore, there will always be scarcity of resources, the key difference between those prosperous and those not so prosperous, the efficiency of resource allocation and utilization, in particular regarding the alternative uses to which they put the resources. These facts apply to every country and to every economy. The problems that confront health systems today are not peculiar, as there have never been enough doctors and nurses and probably will never be, for example. The problems might in fact reflect defects in the allocation and management of scarce healthcare delivery resources now accentuated by the interplay of a variety of other issues in contemporary times, many non-health related, international trade, prices, commerce, globalization, and unemployment, for examples, which are crucial determinants of the wealth of nations, and the well-being of their citizens. To appreciate fully, the interactions between these various issues, including between health issues and between non-health issues, and between health and non-health issues and how they affect healthcare delivery, including the predicament in which many health systems currently wallow, and from which what requires done to extricate them, itself requires contemplative rigor. It is important first, to recognize that the health system is an integral part of the economy and to which economic principles necessarily applies. The imperative stems from the potential for the health industry to affect adversely the rest of the economy left to venture astray. The scarcity of resources in the health industry is evident wherever one looks. For example, no one needs statistical evidence for the shortage of doctors many countries have, or of nurses, and other healthcare professionals, considering for example, the often-long wait times, sometimes even to see their family doctors, healthcare consumers experience even in many developed countries. Nor is the fact that an ever-increasing healthcare spending, which again many countries struggle with, is not only counter-intuitive but also unsustainable. It follows therefore, that it should not take Olympian zeal to convince anyone that the health industry needs to start to optimize the allocation and utilization of its scarce resources. The question then is how. In addressing the challenges that health systems face, policy makers, hospital executive officers, Health Ministry officials, the private sector, even concerned citizens, among other healthcare stakeholders would have to remodel their worldviews of healthcare delivery to factor in the harsh realities of the economic principles that govern life in other domains. The fact of the matter then is that contemporary healthcare delivery is evolving, within the context of our changing world, and it would be naïve if not downright farcical to ignore the potential of the symbiotic dyadic characteristic of the interlocking tango of issues crucial to its outcome.

This realization would for example, highlight the significance of the report in the latest set of government health statistics, *Health United States, 2006*, by the Centers for Disease Control and Prevention (CDC) that 25% of U.S. adults indicate having a daylong pain spell in the past month, and 10% that the pain lasted a year or more[1]. The report released on November 15, 2006 that also showed that infant mortality declined in 2003-04, from 6.9 to 6.8 deaths per 1000 live births, that 11%, and 23% of those 40-50 years old, and 60 years and older, respectively, have diabetes, and that visits to general/family doctors declined from 34% in 1980 to 23% in 2004, is telling. That CDC focused on pain in this year's report is hardly surprising. As the report's lead author, Amy Bernstein noted 'We chose to focus on pain in this report because it is rarely discussed as a condition in and of itself it is mostly viewed as a byproduct of another condition.' She added 'We also chose this topic because the associated costs of pain are posing a great burden on the health care system, and because there are great disparities among different population groups in terms of who suffer from pain.' Considered within a wider perspective, a recent report by the Organization for Economic Cooperation and Development (OECD) highlights the potential ramifications of the burden of disease illness/disability, among reasons for which pain is no doubt paramount, on the overall national economy. The report, *Sickness, Disability, and Work: Breaking the Barriers*, released on November 07, 2006, which analyzed the sickness and disability policies of Norway, Poland and Switzerland noted that large numbers of workers exit the labor market through sickness and disability benefits[2]. The report recommended that these countries do more to reduce these numbers and assist more disabled individuals to return to the labor market. OECD countries in 2004 spent 2.4% of their GDP on sickness and disability, about twice that on unemployment benefit, which itself guzzled 1.3% of GDP that same year. The corresponding figures for sickness/disability for the countries mentioned in the report were over the OECD average, for sickness/disability, between 3% and 5% of GDP, for unemployment, less than the OECD average in all three. The CDC report indicated that low back pain is one of the commonest complaints among Americans, migraine or severe headache, and joint pain, aching or stiffness, others. Indeed, the knee is the joint causing the most pain, hospitalization rates for knee replacement procedures increasing almost 90% between 1992-93 and 2003-04 among seniors 65 years and older. With such potential costs implications of pain not to mention its psychological burden, is it not apposite to explore its dimensions including as did the CDC? Could such explorations not reveal potential areas to address such as sick certificates/absence from work, and benefits issues, in particular as the longer persons are on sickness benefit, the likelier the transition into disability benefit? Would the exploration not eventually result in developing appropriate measures and policies, as OECD suggested the countries mentioned in its report do, to assist those with health issues for example, chronic pain, or disability to return to the labor force? There is no doubt that such measures would improve their financial status, their self-esteem, and help reintegrate them into society, and in the long-term help increase the country's overall productivity hence economic growth and development, which without these measures would not likely materialize, the economy on the other hand, in fact, likely compromised. The varieties of pain reported in the CDC report constitute some of the reasons people transition to disability for examples, low back pain, knee pain, and migraine or severe headaches, which 15% of American adults experience, according to the report. With adults 18-44 years almost thrice as likely as those 65 years and older to report migraines or severe headaches, those likely to go on disability are in the age bracket critical for economic productivity. Should this not be cause for concern? Should we not be seeking ways to reduce the prevalence of pain exploring its roots causes and investing as necessary and even upfront on initiatives, such as health education and promotion, and disease prevention programs, including for example on healthcare information and communications technologies (healthcare ICT) that would facilitate their achievement? Would the benefits in pecuniary, morbidity terms among others that would accrue from this initial investment not outweigh its costs, even if in the long-term? In the U.S. between 1988-94 and 1999-2002, more adults took a narcotic drug to alleviate pain in the past month, 3.2%, and 4.2%, respectively, and the country spent an average of $6,280 per person on health care in 2004, 7% of adults under 65 years indicating they passed up receiving required care for costs reasons in the previous year. What are the implications of an increasing use of narcotics by the public for pain, with the potential for abuse and the subsequent social and other problems? Could these issues not increase health spending, and compromise the overall well-being of society and its economy, individuals most needed for economic productivity for example not receiving the care that they need because they could not afford it? Is it at all possible to prevent these issues by appreciating fully the symbiotic dyadic mentioned above, thus preventing disability in the first place, encouraging those on disability benefits to return to work, even offering employers incentives to cooperate in this effort? Should we not also be discouraging the transition from sickness to disability benefits, and revisiting comprehensively the issues of sick leave and absence from work, among others? Would such all-inclusive appraisals not involve inter-sectoral collaboration with for examples the involvement of health and social security departments, private health insurance, employers, and health, and vocational rehabilitation authorities? Would this collaboration not warrant in-depth evaluation of current resources, their allocation, and utilization, and indeed, an exploration of the approaches to optimizing them for more cost-effective and efficient alternative uses? The answers to these questions and other questions would certainly help in our approach to the economics of healthcare delivery now and in the years ahead that would likely be different in many respects from what we do currently. This would be even more so due to the ongoing need to review the fundamental basis of healthcare delivery, considering what some would term the frenetic pace of progress in the evolution of medical knowledge with implications, sometimes seismically, for shifts in practice paradigms, but also due to the pressures the often-equally profound changes external to it, exert on it.

The point made earlier about initial upfront investment is particular relevant

to the issue of these pressures, and to the reorientation in approach to the economics of healthcare delivery that is in a sense mandatory for addressing the challenges contemporary healthcare delivery faces. Such investments would be necessary for example to address issues of scarcity of healthcare professionals and of their distribution, patently skewed in many countries, most of these professionals concentrated in urban areas, gainsaying the effect of which on accessibility to care by folks living in rural areas clearly unnecessary. Nor would it be, the potential for such investments, in for example, the technologies that could facilitate physician consultation, and treatment, to offset the costs of care and reduce overall health spending while not only ensuring accessibility to care, but also to even more qualitative care as specialist doctors, utilize these technologies to deliver services that some communities hitherto lacked. It is ironical that productivity in these rural communities, which contribute significantly to their countries' economies, should decline because of failure to address these resource-allocation issues, and indeed, those regarding the alternative uses to which we could put these scarce resources, for more efficient and cost-effective operations that would improve, not compromise productivity, and indeed, the entire economy. Paradoxically, the symbiotic dyadic, in its various forms such as the worsening of budgetary and other pressures on the health system of ignoring the issues regarding those living in rural areas, for example, the quality of whose health the lack of accessibility to care depletes, the consequences of which on the overall economy could be devastating, would mandate addressing them. In other words, the new health economics would bear on all aspects of healthcare delivery the principles that govern the efforts of the overall economy to tackle the problems of scarcity and rational resource allocation and utilization crucial for any country's economy to move forward. In an increasingly competitive global arena, it would be rash for any country, health system, or jurisdiction not to acknowledge the potential effects of the shifts in job abroad for example on the its overall economy. It would also be so for such a country not to take the necessary measures to keep the jobs in, or to bring jobs in from abroad in equal or more measure that those abroad need, and for which it has ample expertise and labor. Thus, it is unlikely that any country would thrive in the coming years, which snubs these realities and work arduously to excel in the prevailing dispensation, including paying attention to its health system, the first and most fundamental 'economic' domain that would ensure its competitiveness in the first place in the global markets. It would therefore be necessary to rethink the approach to measuring returns on investments (ROI) in health matters for example, realizing the intangibility of several aspects of healthcare delivery, yet ensuring that judgment on investments is not whimsical. The new economics of health would therefore increasingly be a delicate balancing act but one nonetheless capable of benefiting from rigorous methodology that combines elements of theory and practice in workable measure. It would for example need to be able to recognize the role of process cycle analysis, in alleviating scarcity and in resource allocation/utilization. This process, an exhaustive decomposition and exposition of the various issues involved in the particular outcome of an aspect of healthcare delivery, which would reveal the additional issues and processes that need further decomposing to reveal the appropriate measures necessary to resolve the issues, would be an ongoing exercise for future health systems to survive let alone thrive. This would be so for any health system to achieve the dual healthcare delivery objective (DHDO) of delivering qualitative health services simultaneously reducing health spending, key aspects of an optimal health system essential for ensuring it meets its participatory mandate in interlocking tango mentioned above whose excellence constitutes the main requirement for economic prosperity. It in fact makes intuitive sense to pursue these dual goals. For one, health systems are inherently unstable, due to the factors impinging on them from within, for example, changes in medical knowledge necessitating ongoing re-evaluation of practice, not mention changes to say, accounting systems, such reviews might warrant, such as those that would reflect compliance by agents, say healthcare professionals, to principals' mandate. There are even more unpredictable external factors, both health and non-health related that constantly necessitate changes to the processes that result in healthcare delivery, whose elements therefore would require ongoing reappraisals. The re-evaluation of the effects on the health systems of both these internal and external factors therefore is an important and essentially mandatory activity, were the health system serious about assuring, and in fact improving quality. Considering the spontaneity of the events that sometimes disrupt the status quo of health systems, for example, the potentially cataclysmic changes to a health system that a sudden outbreak of an epidemic due to a previously unknown virus would it not be prudent, to engage in thorough process cycle analyses in anticipation of such changes? Would it not also be so to invest upfront in for example the technological and other solutions that emerge from such analyses, even were their returns on investments not immediate obviously in such domains, in particular, the clinical domains? There is no doubt that such investments could reduce morbidities and mortalities that could escalate healthcare costs, the reduction in costs, and in the psychological burden of disease for example, likely to reduce overall health spending, while in fact improving the quality of healthcare delivery. The new health economics therefore needs to embrace the concept of the dual healthcare delivery objectives (DHDO) and adjust its mechanics to addressing healthcare delivery issues within the parameters of the concept, a reorientation that could jettison certain elements of the current approaches to the health sector by the economics zeitgeist. The debate over the benefits of catastrophic health insurance coverage vis-à-vis comprehensive coverage would become moot for example, not doing otherwise. Yet, from the fundamental wellspring of the need for access to care by all would emanate issues that highlight the symbiotic dyadic that renders such a discussion redundant. In other words, these issues place the healthcare consumer not at the fringe but at the center of the healthcare delivery universe, literally. This makes providing access to healthcare by as many as who could contribute to the economic prosperity of a country being and remaining in good health critical to achieve. Does this mean escalating healthcare costs, likely not, for the simple reason of the elimination, or the potential for so doing, in the long-term, the adverse selection that does the opposite of access to care for many, essentially excluding them also from making required contribution to the workforce, and to the country's economy. This again, highlights the point about the need for rethinking approaches to health economics, coupled in particular with the benefits accruable from investments in such provision upfront, as with the case of the rural residents mentioned earlier including the costs offset later by the reduction in illness-related costs, and by the overall increase in the country's economic output. National competitiveness is more important in present-day global economic milieu than it has ever been, depends on a variety of factors and explains marked differences such as those between the rich and poor countries, and even among each group, some of these factors, relatively minute, or so they appear relative to others in either boosting or hindering economic productivity. As every economic sector should, and which indeed, is in their best interests to do, the health industry needs to re-examine how it conducts its business. Thus, in ensuring that the health industry pays its dues in boosting national competitiveness, the requirement for fundamental changes in orientation toward healthcare delivery explains why for example rather than allow individuals to spend precious time waiting for an appointment to see their GP, Alberta,

Canada, is introducing a scheme whereby pharmacists would be able to prescribe some medications. Would this measure not reduce morbidities and perhaps even mortalities, the ethico-moral implications of not doing otherwise clear, not to mention its potential to help the province achieve the dual healthcare delivery objectives, and to improve the residents' overall health, hence the province's economic productivity, hence contribution to the country's competitiveness on the global economic stage? Does this measure not exemplify the alternative uses to which putting scarce resources would alleviate scarcity and enhance economic growth and sustainable development? Would for example, besides training the pharmacists that opt for the program, establishing real-time communication link between them and the GPs, or other doctors that treat the healthcare consumers, not enhance further the quality of service provision by all the healthcare providers, with the availability at the point of care (POC) vital information that they might need in delivering care? Would the investments in these technologies, some that might in fact be substantial, for example, by the GP in a complete suite of electronic medical records (EMR) technologies, not be worth the while in the long-term, considering the benefits to the patient, and the costs-savings this would engender, among other benefits? For example, with the patient being increasingly at the center of the healthcare delivery universe, would the enhanced value proposition of the healthcare providers able to communicate and share patient information in the is manner not result in increased patronage, hence profitability? These benefits would accrue regardless of the funding of the health system, incidentally, which underscores the point made earlier about catastrophic or comprehensive coverage, or indeed that between publicly or privately funded health systems.

That the health system is an integral part of the economic system in both

settings is not in doubt, nor is the need for it to contribute positively to the economy, the question being essentially the modalities involved and the tactical and operational maneuverings warranted and to what extent regarding such contributions. It is thus that, and it is already happening, a hospital in Canada, would need to justify its existence increasingly in the new dispensation, or face the prospects of closure, much as any in the U.S., or the U.K. This is despite differences in health funding approaches in these countries, in which incidentally both public and private funds play significant roles, but to varying extents. A hospital therefore in Canada for example, would also need to enhance its value proposition to retain patronage, hence for continued viability more so in for example Quebec, where private and public health system run in parallel, but also in other provinces, even for services Medicare covers, as the consumer still has the choice of receiving the services elsewhere. Even if they sought those services at their own expenses elsewhere because for example, they did not want to wait for so long to receive them in a hospital that is not enhancing its services, could prices of the services not fall sufficiently to deplete the hospital's clientele to threaten its survivability? Even if such hospitals then had to close down a surgical wing, could it not eventually have to close down in its entirety and could this not have not happened simply enhancing its value proposition by an investment that might seem at first unprofitable? Besides, would the hospital by allowing the moribund process to materialize in termination, not have denied perhaps a small number of patrons who could not afford seeking services elsewhere access to needed care, creating costs for the health system, doing the exact opposite of what it should in contributing to economic progress? This explains why even with publicly funded systems, that the healthcare consumer is central to healthcare delivery, which would become increasingly as part of the convergence of efforts, albeit sometimes without even realizing it, toward ensuring the health sector plays its role effectively and efficiently in the progress of the overall economy, would inevitably necessitate new approaches to health economics. It would necessitate for example conceptualizing healthcare delivery, as a number of processes that could hampered or facilitated, become crucial rate limiting steps in the care delivery enterprise. It would therefore be necessary to conduct process cycle analyses to determine the effectiveness and efficiency, even viability of these processes, to ensure they do not clog the entire healthcare delivery enterprise, ensuring which might involve implementing solutions including healthcare information technologies, with costs implications. Indeed, the new health economics would involve consideration of issues such as initiating novel and improving existing approaches to reduce transactions costs, both ex-ante, such as contract preparation, and related issues, and ex-post, for example contractor monitoring and sanctions implementation for contractual breaches, in healthcare delivery, besides process facilitation by these technologies. It would also involve assuring accountability, and in particular devising the most context-appropriate relationships between and aligning the goals of principals and agents in the variety of transactions involved in healthcare delivery. As Paul (1992)[3] noted, there are three principal ways to ensure accountability namely exit, shifting demand to another provider; voice, democratic mechanisms at play and; hierarchy, system assurance of accountability, and each would play an increasing role in the future of healthcare delivery. For example, exit and voice mechanisms underline the increasing role healthcare consumers would play and how their ability to choose, hence exit undesirable services, would influence the entire healthcare delivery enterprise and its potential to contribute positively to the economy. The new health economics would also be part of the process of refashioning entrenched notions such as dictated at least in part by the pervasive information asymmetry within the health sector, regarding the ability of the average healthcare consumer to make the informed choices capable of improving accountability. This would be in keeping with the need for concerted efforts by all stakeholders to contribute to the changes required for the health system to achieve the dual healthcare delivery objectives, in which they are especially interested, tethering as it were, around the core tenets of economics. It would therefore be necessary to appreciate the need for promoting the widespread diffusion of healthcare information and communication technologies as a part of the efforts to rectify this information asymmetry, including offering incentives to doctors and other healthcare professionals to acquire and implement these technologies. Not even scale economies should deter the quest to make the healthcare consumers more capable of making rational choices regarding their health, and health jurisdictions in addition to promoting the technologies that could facilitate health information dissemination, should establish appropriate boards, community relations committees, and organizations that offer healthcare consumers avenues for expressing opinions on service delivery and other issues. These measures are in keeping with not just the requirements of a patient-centered healthcare delivery model, they are important to making the model work, and the model functioning efficiently to the health system meeting its obligations to the entire economy. Part of the health system being able to achieve this goal is to make the right choices in its allocation of its doctors and nurses for example, and the utilization of its lab resources, and its medications. That the healthcare consumer is at the center of healthcare delivery also helps make this happen, because at least in part they also have a stake in making rational choices regarding healthcare providers, the services they provide, including the lab tests they order, and the medications they prescribe. This underscores the need for adopting this broader-based perspective of healthcare delivery that emphasizes the interface of the processes involved with other non-health related processes and issues, all operating in tandem toward achieving the same goal, which essentially is national economic prosperity. An important dimension of the role healthcare ICT would play in the achievement of the DHDO hence of the contributions of the health sector to the overall economy besides its specific symbiotic dyadic with healthcare delivery that could itself transform either , in turn both by each other, as progress in one feeds into and modifies the other, is instructive. This dimension accentuates the potential for an appreciation and adoption of the viewpoint stated above on the pace of not just the quest to achieve the DHDO, but also to ensure its contribution to economic growth and development considering the changing dynamics of world prosperity and the increasing competitiveness on the global arena not just between businesses but also countries. China for example, is at present the largest exporter of ICT goods and progressively ascending the value chain, the Indian ICT industry also doing quite well, firms adopting global strategies, with offices in the US., Canada, and Europe, from where they also recruit software engineers, underlining the point made earlier about the need to offer the world enhanced value propositions. Experts are in fact wondering whether these countries could sustain the pace at which they are going currently, if they could have enough local engineering/management expertise to compete favorably on the global stage, and if developed economies, many flustered by the flight of jobs due to outsourcing to cheaper labor-markets in less developed countries, could meet the resulting challenges. Would it therefore be necessary for example, for developed countries to create the enabling environment, one with healthy and productive citizens, for the education and training in the expertise needed by the ever-growing ICT industry, including healthcare ICT that countries, such as China and India need but lack, or of which they do not or would not eventually have enough? Would investing in the appropriate solutions, including the healthcare ICT that would help improve access to health services for example, and that would help achieve the DHDO not therefore be apt under these circumstances the return on such investments evident even if in later years, not just on the health system, but on the country's overall economy? China surpassed the

United States in 2004 becoming the world's number one exporter of information and communications technology (ICT) goods for examples, mobile phones, notebooks, and digital cameras[4]. China exported US$180 billion worth of ICT goods that year, versus US$149 billion by the U.S., in contrast to 2003, when the latter led with US$137 billion, China's, US$123 billion. China's portion of total (imports/exports) global trade in ICT goods were US$35 billion, US$234 billion, and US$329 billion in 1996, 2003, and 2004, respectively, versus the U.S's US$230 billion, US$301 billion, and US$375 billion during the same years, respectively. Would it not be necessary for the U.S., for example to hike its exports of ICT goods to China, to rectify the trade imbalance between the two countries in favor of the latter, with huge Chinese trade surpluses in computer & related equipment? Is this not the more urgent in particular as the data from the OECD indicate that China is trading more with other Asian countries, from where it now sources most of its computer chips for example, with resultant fall in ICT imports not just to China but also to the entire region from European Union (EU) countries and the U.S[5]? With China the leading ICT goods exporter to the U.S, 27% of all U.S ICT imports in 2004 from there, versus just 10% in 2000, the country's ICT trade surplus with the U.S, US$34 billion in 2004, with the EU, US$27 billion, could the healthcare delivery/healthcare ICT symbiotic dyadic not help rectify the situation? There is no doubt about the potential of the in tandem feedback process between these two to stimulate the development of innovative ICT products/service mixes with immense sales potential in China, in other Asian countries, and indeed, worldwide. This only further highlights the need for re-conceptualizing healthcare delivery to embrace its wider role in national economic growth. This would no doubt energize the creative potential of the enormous talent and expertise in the U.S., and indeed, other countries that would result in novel technologies that would improve healthcare delivery, cost-effectively too and that would be marketable even in other countries would emerge. The implications of developments in healthcare delivery therefore include stimulating the emergence of new technologies to meet the challenges these developments spawn, the new technologies not just solving the emergent problems, but also creating opportunities for equally novel healthcare-delivery models, the symbiotic dyadic that ensues, with wider implications for the entire economy. Would it not be necessary therefore for the new health economics to embrace the need to invest in these technologies? Is it any wonder then that U.S Health and Human Services Secretary Michael Leavitt said November 17, 2006, that a competitive healthcare market based on quality and cost savings to the healthcare consumer is the only way to change the U.S. health system? He was speaking at a summit, "Implementing Healthcare Transparency". His audience was hundreds of employers to reinforce efforts to improve the U.S. economy via healthcare transformation, based on President Bush's healthcare transparency plan, which an August 2006 executive order mandated[6], and to which Federal healthcare programs, for examples Medicare, the Veterans Affairs health system and the Federal Employees Health Benefit Program must adhere in 2007. Leavitt rightly considered healthcare IT the key to instituting "value-driven healthcare, " and as he also rightly noted, interoperability and being able to communicate and share quality, outcome and cost data will fuel the consumer-driven healthcare market, including moderating care pricing, as competition among care givers within a fully operational market economy would drive prices down.

The U.S. healthcare market makes up 16% of the gross national product,

hence offers immense opportunities for market forces to operate and manifestly too. By embracing value-driven transparent healthcare, healthcare stakeholders would be contributing to the full expression of these forces, to the benefit of all. Companies should, therefore, be seeking qualitative health services, and healthcare providers offering them, the role healthcare information and communication technologies would play in the process, quite likely significant. Indeed, Leavitt predicted that within 2 years, there would be in the U.S., quality and cost competition within local markets for some healthcare procedures, that value-driven healthcare would be the benchmark of care within five years, and that within ten years, would be countrywide, that based on the Bush plan for transparency. The Secretary's predictions underline the momentum of the evolution of healthcare in the country being crucial and its ties with the markets and the country's economy overall being substantial, progress in the increasing interplay of the two is unlikely stoppable. This perhaps puts the recent decision by America's Health Insurance Plans revealed on November 13, 2006, in its true perspective[7]. The "roadmap for reform" aims to expand health insurance coverage to include the over 40 million uninsured Americans. The roadmap, titled *Access for All Americans*, would enhance current public programs, and engage state and federal legislators, the public, and private sectors. Electronic health records (EHR) would contribute to reduction in healthcare costs required to support the plan, which again attests to the point made earlier about the significant role of healthcare ICT in the evolution of healthcare delivery, indeed, not just in the U.S., but also elsewhere worldwide. Thus, part of the new healthcare economics would be determining the nature, extent, and pace of the implementation of these technologies and programs in relation to a country's economy, and its growth and development, as for example George Halvorson, chairman-elect of AHIP's board of directors suggested for *Access for All Americans* that it would require phased implementation. Thus, expanding access first to cover all children within 3 years, and 95% of adults within a decade, would facilitate the achievement of a realistic approach to the program, according to AHIP, which reckons that full implementation of the proposal would cost the federal government roughly $300 billion over a 10-year span[7]. This means that with President Bush seeking $200 billion for healthcare spending, AHIP would,

$10 billion annually over 10 years, which it is uncertain how to raise but stressed not so doing, hence not paying attention to the problems of access to care, would be disastrous. Indeed, signs of this are already evident with an average insured family currently paying about $1,000 of its yearly premium toward covering care to the uninsured, payment for which it would not receive any compensation[7]. Rightly, so, AHIP considers disease prevention, in particular of chronic diseases, as a key aspect of the cost reduction that would subsidize expanded coverage for more Americans, again, difficult, if not indeed, impossible to gainsay the importance of deploying efficiently and cost-effectively, the appropriate healthcare information and communication technologies in this regard. AHIP wants to expand the State Children's Health Insurance Program and Medicaid, to cover all uninsured children from low-income families, and all uninsured adults with incomes less than the federal poverty level, respectively. It also wants the establishment of a new tax-free healthcare account for families and individuals to utilize for healthcare coverage and that of a child healthcare tax credit for working families, as well as a new incentive grant program to help states expand access to healthcare. No doubt, not the American health system, or indeed, any other could afford to ignore the issue of access to healthcare nor in fact, that of ensuring the delivery of qualitative health services cost-effectively, in effect to ignore the dual healthcare delivery objectives (DHDO.) The aspect of quality is so important it is at the core of achieving the DHDO, and would therefore warrant utmost attention. It would thus be necessary to focus on ways to achieve it, for example as HHS Secretary Leavitt also noted on November 13, 2006, that of establishing a scorecard that stipulates how well a hospital or doctor performs regarding patient care, and their pricing, which he asserted, could assist in transforming health care in the country. The Secretary in fact plans to encourage private insurers and employers to help develop and utilize such a scorecard to help the healthcare consumer make educated choices regarding healthcare providers, services, and prices. There is also no doubt that healthcare ICT has an important role to play in the success of such scorecards, enabling the delivery, efficiently and cost-effectively, the information required by the healthcare consumer to make such decisions, the need for their widespread implementation by all relevant stakeholders, self-evident. In fact, employers and insurance firms provide significant portions of health benefits in the U.S, hence it is in their best interests to seek to be able to continue to do so, less expensively, yet without compromising the quality of healthcare delivery, in other words, to strive to achieve the DHDO too. The healthcare consumer also would save substantial out-of-pocket costs making the right healthcare delivery choices, hence in their interests to pursue the DHDO. By implementing the relevant healthcare information and communication technologies, both payers and payees would be able to exchange valuable information that would ensure the delivery of high quality health services and that would reduce costs, ultimately. Rating care quality would be an important aspect of the entire quality assurance process, and EHR would play a key role in this regard, helping to keep tab on each procedure, prescription, and diagnosis, facilitating an audit process. This would, among others help inform future policy, including measures to consolidate on quality gains, and improve it where lacking, all of which would help achieve the dual healthcare delivery objectives, at various levels, and ultimately at the national level. Government would play a key supportive role in the process, which itself would encourage active participation of the private sector, and of the healthcare consumer. Considering that, most surveys have indicated healthcare to be consistently among the top five major concerns of Americans, most actually dissatisfied with the health system's status, soliciting support from which would be less arduous as it seem might at first in achieving the DHDO. As in the U.S., healthcare is important to the majority of peoples all over the world. It is as if peoples intuitively understand the need to be healthy and strong to be happy and productive. Except for a relatively few persons that for some reasons do not or no longer consider life worth living, individuals society incidentally also has obligations to ensure receive the needed medical and other types of assistance many such persons need, it would take an effort literally, for death to occur in many other than instantaneously by accident or otherwise. In other words, most peoples would rather live, and would struggle not to die. Actually, many that die, do not have to, at least not at the time they did, were they to receive the healthcare that they needed before matters got out of hands, literally. That the emotional loss incurred by those they left behind not to mention the economic loss of their say, palliative care, were avoidable costs that could directly and indirectly increase health spending by their health jurisdiction, would be an understatement but one nonetheless worthy of attention, and correction. Thus, every health jurisdiction should, as a matter of moral and economic expediency attempt to achieve the dual healthcare delivery objectives, even if the pressures internal and external to it, and over which it has little if any control also mandate it does. Compliance with these mandates by health systems would ensure the delivery of qualitative health services that would in turn reduce morbidities and mortalities, hence healthcare costs, and spending. The underlying changes in the mechanisms and processes of healthcare delivery that this would involve constitute the ingredients for the evolution that health economics would undergo along with the healthcare delivery and healthcare information and communication dyadic. In other words, we are going to see health systems worldwide in the coming years essentially compelled to make the necessary reforms possible that would result or at least lead them in the direction of achieving the dual healthcare delivery objectives. Health systems would have to seek ways to improve the quality of service delivery or risk oblivion in effect as the economies within which they operate groan under soaring healthcare bills, threatening other areas of economic activities, in particular private sector businesses, pressures on the health systems to perform increasing in intensity as a result. These developments would be irrespective of the funding system of healthcare in these jurisdictions, considering the ties between the health system and the other aspects of a country's economy. Would it matter the funding system of a health system for example the fact that obesity could knock economic output as brutally as malnutrition, which depletes up to 3% of production in poor countries? The World Health Organization (WHO) notes obesity has tripled in the past twenty years, and that one in 10 children and one in five adults would be obese in Europe and Central Asia in another four years were action not taken. This, again, underlines the key role healthcare information and communication technologies could play in not just the health but also the wealth of nations. Adult obesity incurs presently about 6% of health costs in the WHO's European region, including Central Asia, according to WHO, in France in 1992, costing $12.1 billion in just direct costs, obesity/overweight costing California, $22 billion, in both direct and indirect costs in 2000. Obesity being associated with a number of diseases such as diabetes, some chronic in nature, would also reduce the life span in many individuals, which overall would deplete the labor force and compromise a country's economy that ignores these issues, men in England projected for example to live five less years the current prevalence of obesity not addressed. Interestingly, obesity/overweight is not unique to developed countries, and developing countries also have increasing overweight/obese populations, hence obesity is no longer peculiar to the rich, some say the reverse might even be true with the escalation of 'junk food' among the poor, in France obesity five times more prevalent among low-than high-income groups, for example. Others assert that both the rich and the poor are now obese in most countries, the rich due to their increasingly docile life style. The problem is that the economic consequences of obesity on the poorer, developing countries, which already face enormous depletion of their human resources by infections of various sorts, including HIV/AIDS, would likely be more catastrophic. Hence, these countries, perhaps even more urgently need to devise means, including the massive deployment of the healthcare information and communication technologies best suited to their contexts, by which to achieve the DHDO.

Among other measures therefore would be the need to encourage people to consume healthier food and to exercise, both of which healthcare ICT, would help facilitate. Some have even suggested the use of inducements, including economic for this purpose, for example, taxes on pop, and in some jurisdictions, for example, in Saskatchewan, the province is considering legislation that would enable it sue tobacco companies, to receive compensation for the costs to the province of treating smoking related illnesses, which costs it over $145 million dollars annually.

These issues show that not only is it important for health jurisdictions to

address the issues of qualitative healthcare delivery but also to ensure that they deliver these services cost-effectively and efficiently. Regardless of the nature of the funding for the health jurisdiction therefore, the need for measures such as accountability, transparency, efficiency, effectiveness, and responsiveness, among others become paramount. Part of the tasks of the new health economics would be ensuring adherence to these principles, without which it would not only be difficult to effect the required changes to facilitate the achievement of the DHDO, but also to implement new measures, rules, and regulations, that would help in achieving these important goals. In other words, the activities health jurisdictions engage in need to be clear in all aspects to the public, including the benefits derivable from the health expenditure funded with public funds. It would be much easier for example for health jurisdictions to cultivate public trust in its projects were such projects conducted in the most transparent manner, the public appreciating the efforts of its health jurisdiction to improve health services while curtailing health spending. The health jurisdiction or government would need this trust, which essentially is capital it could later invest in new projects, without much difficulty or opposition from the public, in particular if it also made its activities transparent to the public. This would make the ongoing and necessary adaptation to changes within and without the health system crucial to its survival, ensuring budgetary consolidation, and the most efficient allocation and utilization of scarce resources possible, including coupling these to outcomes, in particular, to the most cost-effective and efficient. These adaptations predicate on the health jurisdictions' abilities to innovate and to be flexible in applying novel ideas, management approaches, and technologies, in particular the healthcare information and communication technologies that would improve the variety of processes involved in healthcare delivery. Health jurisdictions would also need to explore alternative uses to deploy scarce resources for utmost efficiency and the generation of most benefits, including promoting public/private sector partnerships, and other inter-sectoral alliances, including outsourcing services, to moderate transaction costs, including in fact reducing them, simultaneously achieving the best services for its resource input. The new economics of healthcare delivery would therefore need to be able to promote the means by which health jurisdictions could achieve these goals, and operate at enhanced levels, creating better opportunities for them to achieve the DHDO. With the healthcare consumer at the center of the healthcare delivery enterprise as we noted earlier, a position that the achievement of the DHDO, and indeed, the evolution of systems, including the health system, worldwide mandates, the need for dialogue with the public is critical to the success of efforts to achieve the DHDO, and other healthcare delivery goals. This calls for the establishment of consultative assemblies/bodies, and for educating healthcare consumers on their functions, and on how they could contribute to the success of their operations, which among others would facilitate efforts by health jurisdictions, and governments to refocus resource allocation and utilization around outcomes. As noted earlier, this most crucial consideration in economics would be the single most important guiding principle as contemporary healthcare delivery transitions into the future, investments in the means to improve outcomes, such as healthcare information and communication technologies, without increasing health spending, likely to increase as resources remain scarce, if not in fact increasingly scarcer. It would be increasingly evident to health jurisdictions for example, the need or otherwise to outsource radiological services and others to external health jurisdictions, including outside the country, to alleviate surgical wait times due to the shortage of radiologists in that particular health jurisdiction, being one consideration perhaps among others faced with such issues. Several issues would need reappraisal in the new health economics, for example patient safety, medical errors, narcotic scams, defensive medicine, repeat lab testing, and so on that have important implications for healthcare costs escalating, hence health spending. These issues also bring to the fore the need to invest in healthcare information and communication technologies upfront as these technologies, even if the returns on these investments do not come until much later down the road, have the potential to help address the issues successfully, and to achieve the dual healthcare delivery objectives. They could also help in devising and implementing the appropriate physician reimbursement system for the particular health jurisdiction. Thus, they could help ease the concerns of many regarding the pay-for-performance model for example, by making the evaluation of the contributions of different physicians involved in the care of the healthcare consumer more objective and readily measurable. These technologies could therefore help avoid controversies regarding billings, in particular with the healthcare consumer also able, via say personal health records (PHR) technologies, to track services received and the payments made from each of the healthcare providers. They would also help promote the evolution of novel health services delivery approaches, for examples, electronic consultations, which would streamline service provision in many instances, and optimize resource utilization, saving the healthcare consumer time and money, as they do the health system. These technologies would make it easier to determine payment for such services, and would facilitate payments for some services via credit cards for example. There is no doubt about the immense benefits of healthcare information and communication technologies and the need to promote their widespread applications in the delivery of health services. The point in fact is that we would increasingly have little if any choice in so doing, the consequences for the health system of the alternatives too stark to even contemplate. The consumer-centric orientation of health services that seems increasingly pervasive in the developed world would increasingly also involve patients being involved more in matters of their health, including financially. This would require the healthcare consumer to be more discerning and accountable. Many would certainly like to be but that they do not have the right information to enable them achieve these goals is another major issue that we need to confront as we manipulate the health system to meet the demands of the new health economics, in this instance the efficient and judicious use of scarce healthcare delivery resources. This essentially would be in the best interests of the healthcare consumer, as his or her expenditures on health services would decrease, yet the quality of the services obtained would not. It might be easier to spend someone else's money, but what healthcare consumers that abhor making contributions to the funds used in their care fail to realize is that the money is in fact theirs, not someone else's. It is therefore still in their best interests to spend it judiciously and cost effectively, lest they risk paying more taxes, higher insurance premiums, and having less resources for the provision of other essential services that society needs. A more discerning healthcare consumer would thus, not pay frivolous visits to the doctor or make unnecessary complaints once there. The new health economics would make it unlikely that the doctor in turn would order or repeat tests that contribute little if any to the treatment of the patient, or the patient to accept without question direct-to-consumer advertising, which in 2000 added $2.6 billion to U.S. spending on drugs[8]. The population in many developed countries is aging, and the pool of doctors, particularly doctors in primary is dwindling, 20% Internal medicine residents in the U.S., keen to go into primary 20% in 2005 compared to 54% in 1998[9], many of the baby-boomers expected to retire in another five years themselves doctors. There is no doubt therefore, about the potential looming crisis in healthcare delivery, particularly at the primary care level, in these countries. In the U.S., the Current Procedural Terminology (CPT) codes ostensibly compensate complex decision making, the sort many primary care physicians, who treat the chronically ill and the elderly many with multiple health problems, encounter, at least those that do not fall for the temptation to see more in less time in order to make enough money. Clearly, this is a major issue requiring urgent attention, devising the appropriate remuneration for primary care physicians, as part of the efforts to ensure the continuity of service provision in the first place at that service delivery level. There are of course varieties of potential choices to make in tackling these problems, including those that would require a significant healthcare ICT input. As mentioned earlier, these technologies make it easier to measure the quality of service delivery and in the reimbursements of doctors and other healthcare providers, but they could also help improve service provision to underserved areas, via telehealth for example. They could, also help reduce the need for defensive medicine, by promoting the use of evidence-based practice for example, and in reforming tort laws in countries such as the U.S., where these laws no doubt constitute major hindrances to efforts to reduce health spending. Regardless of whether we put a cap on damages or seek to address the root causes of the problems, tort reform clearly results in a fall in insurance premiums and doctors moving back to underserved areas as the example of Texas shows[10]. Such reforms would complement efforts to benchmark practice mentioned above, which the use of the appropriate healthcare ICT would ensure, hence the need to promote the adoption of these technologies by doctors and other healthcare professionals. The point here is that at the core of the new health economics would be the utilization of the information and communication technologies that could help reallocate scarce health services resources in ways that could make the effects of the scarcity less traumatic, if at all to the health system. In addition, however, and this is a key point as well, making the health system run effectively and efficiently, which achieving the dual healthcare delivery objectives that the widespread implementation of these technologies would help achieve, would also help improve other domains of a country's economy, and indeed, its entire economy. In effect, the evolution of healthcare delivery would ensure that the new health economics provide us with the tools and methodologies to achieve these goals. The forces that would interplay to direct the evolution of the health services in many countries would be such that scarce healthcare resources might even become scarcer, creating such pressures on health systems to justify their very existence essentially that the need to take more seriously and apply the principles of economics to healthcare delivery would be undeniable. This in itself is not only long overdue, but critical, and would bode well for health services delivery worldwide, on the one hand, and might just be the reality sharpener that many countries, particularly in the developing countries need to brace up and improve not just their economies but in doing so, the welfare of their peoples. It is clear that the links between health and the rest of the economy would begin to influence the shape and pace of events in domains traditionally considered non-health, but which the emerging reality indicate are rather 'health-extensions,' with potential positive consequences for us all.

References

1. Available at: http://www.cdc.gov/od/oc/media/pressrel/r061115.htm
Accessed on November 18, 2006

2. Available at:
http://www.oecd.org/document/32/0,2340,en_2649_201185_37635040_1_1_1_1,
00.html Accessed on November 18, 2006

3. Paul, S. (1992) Accountability in public service: exit, voice, and control. *World
Development* 20(7): 1047-60
4. Available at:
http://www.oecd.org/document/8/0,2340,en_2649_201185_35833096_1_1_1_1,0
0.html Accessed on November 19, 2006

5. Available at:
http://www.oecd.org/document/60/0,2340,en_2649_201185_35834236_1_1_1_1,
00.html Accessed on November 19, 2006

6. Available at: http://www.healthcareitnews.com/printStory.cms?id=5939
Accessed on November 25, 2006

7. Available at: http://www.healthcareitnews.com/printStory.cms?id=5921
Accessed on November 25, 2006

8. Kaiser Family Foundation. Impact of direct-to-consumer advertising on
prescription drug spending. Available at: http://www.kff.org/rxdrugs/6084-
index.cfm Accessed November 25, 2006.

9. Terry K. Where's primary care headed? Med Econ. 2006; 83:74-76.

10. Gingrich N, Gill JT. Prodigal state. The Wall Street Journal. May 4, 2006. Available at: http://www.opinionjournal.com/cc/?id=110008328 Accessed November 25, 2006.

The Continuing Evolution

Of

Health Insurance

Access of healthcare remains a key healthcare delivery issue in many

countries, as does that the mechanisms involved continue to be contentious. Not
many would dismiss millions not being able to access needed health services as
trivial. Nor would most persons likely contend that consensus on the many
issues relating to health insurance and its mechanisms, comes easy. In fact, the

challenges that providing qualitative health services to all pose continue to multiply in numbers and complexity in most countries. Among other health-related reasons, this is due to the changing and sometimes 'disruptive' disease prevalence and patterns in an increasingly linked global milieu and the ostensibly frenetic pace of progress in medical knowledge with resulting information glut often in disparate, disjointed, and isolated domains, even within the same health jurisdiction. There are also non-health related reasons for the worsening challenges, and include increasing budgetary pressures on health systems to curtail soaring health spending, issues with employer-sponsored healthcare coverage, developments in the insurance industry, and in government policies and programs on health insurance, and in fact in other, non-insurance domains, but with spillover effects on health and health insurance. In the U.S., for example, the projected doubling of expenditures on three key areas of entitlements for baby-boomers due to retire in another five years, namely Medicare, Medicaid, and Social Security, $1 trillion to $2 trillion in 2005, and 2015, respectively[1], has some wondering from where the money to pay the retired seniors would come. This would no doubt heighten calls by many for cutting back on federal spending, which would increase pressure on the health system to rein in its seeming runaway health spending, with potential consequences for all aspects of healthcare delivery in the country. Such calls have included in countries such as the U.K., those for having a variety of healthcare suppliers and assorted healthcare funding models, for example social insurance, as obtained in countries such as France, Germany, and Switzerland. This is as opposed to the tendency to hike taxes for example, to fund healthcare, which many argue the public not only generally dislikes, but also tends to hurt the economy in the end[2]. These fiscal issues bring squarely to the fore, the debate ongoing in many developed countries regarding the most appropriate way to fund healthcare, proponents of public, private, and mixed funding models pitched against one another, an important aspect of the debate the catastrophic versus comprehensive health insurance coverage. This in turn reveals the argument by some for the need to revisit conceptually what insurance really means as perhaps the starting point in any consideration of modifying its underlying mechanisms to make coverage more affordable hence reach more persons, in particular in countries such as the U.S., where there is no universal health insurance coverage. The lack of consensus on various health insurance issues reflects the ongoing evolution of the concept of health insurance. It concerns for example, whether it is better to have all fund it, or just workers and employers, as with a social insurance system, which critics deem simply a work tax, and inequitable, affording contributors much more leverage over treatment, and whose problems the French health system's 10 billion euro deficit in 2004, typified[2]. Many would prefer the strict use of insurance in healthcare to mean protection of financial assets against the atypical, random, catastrophic event, as used in other types of insurance[3]. Yet, most persons seek coverage for precisely the opposite reasons, which technically is not insurance, since those atypical catastrophic events are indeed, rare, which is partly why many contest the use of and the wisdom in the term for universal health coverage. That health insurance in its customary practice simply is a financial mechanism with which the insured buys in into an ever more exorbitant system of healthcare delivery suggests that the critical outcome of our conceptual redefinition of health insurance should be making the health system more inexpensive. What role could the widespread implementation of healthcare information and communication technologies (ICT) play in this regard, and should universal health insurance not be emphasizing disease prevention, health promotion, and wellness for examples, more so in our increasingly consumer-directed healthcare delivery world, with the healthcare consumer requiring ever more high-deductible plans to ensure receiving treatment in particular for chronic illnesses? Should these measures not be even more urgent considering the pressures, current and imminent on health systems threatening their ability to survival let alone prosper, not to mention the intricacies of how the health system and a nation's economy intimately coalesce, and synergistically? Some have suggested that the U.S., federal government for example, terminating, devolving to the states, or privatizing some programs could save the country up to $380 billion yearly, the value in 2005, $450 billion calculated on the basis of the Congressional Budget Office baseline discretionary spending's growth rate[4]. In Canada, the recent update on the country's economy by Conservative Finance Minister Jim Flaherty appeared to critics though prudent fiscally, socially indifferent. This is a vague reference to the update's focus on smaller government, and tax cuts, the largesse from the latter not showered on health and social welfare and environmental programs, even with new funding for education in such high profile areas as biotechnology and assistance for motivated individuals to break away from welfare[5]. This is not to mention the ruckus provoked by the plan's goal of eliminating Canada's total government 'net debt' by 2021, all future government surpluses used to pay down debt, the money saved on interest payments converted into tax cuts for its citizens, the ambiguity of 'net debt', the starting point for its critique. Further, many remain uncertain about how the federal government plans to eliminate the $481-billion 'federal debt,' if equivalent to the 'total government net debt,' which includes provincial debt and pension plans. The complications involved in the federal government attempting to pressure for example, the provinces and territories to act on these debts, and the potential effects of precipitous actions by which latter to clear them up for health and social welfare programs, self-evident. This is the more so as any future government in the country would have to raise taxes to increase spending, not able to use surpluses, with potential trickle-down implications for Medicare, which though administered by the provinces and territories, receives substantial federal funding. With the country's population aging, and its baby-boomers preparing for retirement in a few years, the implications of the imminent budget crunch for health services provision could not be starker. In other words, health insurance would, via its mechanisms even in a country the bulk of which the public funds, be covering an increasingly unaffordable healthcare delivery system, particularly if provinces and territories devolved more coverage areas to individuals' out-of-pocket coverage via private health insurance firms. Here again, we see the need to make the health system more affordable, in this instance for all payers, provincial/territorial governments, and Canadians alike. Thus, regardless of the health system's funding model, the effects of the changing milieu in which healthcare delivery occurs, driven by both health and non-health related factors, intrinsic and extrinsic to the health system, motorize the evolution of health insurance in all its ramifications. The transience of the changes constitute the fuel for the adjustments the in tandem operations of the health/insurance dyadic demand. In other words, we need to begin to conceptualize and on an ongoing basis thus modify our conceptualizations of health insurance and the most effective ways for its mechanisms to work in keeping with the mandates of the multiplicity of factors impinging on healthcare delivery vis-à-vis the prevailing health and insurance zeitgeist. Indeed, pursuant to the goals the imperative of healthcare delivery transition that we would see in the years ahead, these re-conceptualizations would not need enforcing, as they would flow along with the changes taking place in the health system. For example, the increasing focus on preventive rather than curative healthcare would influence considerations of adverse selections, and no doubt those of the types of insurance coverage and the pricing of insurance premiums available and to whom. Nonetheless, this requires active efforts on our part to ensure that all parties benefit from the encounter, as we do not want to see the health insurance industry collapse for example, nor do we want the health system to do so. Such efforts require an in-depth understanding of the varieties of transactional processes involved in all aspects of healthcare delivery, ranging from access to care to physician reimbursement, among others, the analyses of which processes would reveal additional processes and the mechanisms for modifying them including facilitating some, even excluding others. These analyses, specifically process cycle analyses, would start with an exploration of determined issues of relevance to a particular country or health jurisdiction. They would comprise a variety of decompositions and expositions crucial to achieving the dual healthcare delivery objectives (DHDO) of qualitative healthcare delivery simultaneously reducing health spending, which the complex interplay of factors in achieving would benefit all parties involved in the many transactions culminating in healthcare delivery.

That the DHDO imperative would be difficult if not impossible for the health insurance industry to ignore is evident in developments in various healthcare delivery domains, as for example, in the U.S., where policy debates continue on the contributions of long-term care (LTC) spending to Medicaid's overall spending. In this regard, a recent report that not only is Medicaid's LTC users spending a third of the agency's budget, but that the picture is even much larger, 52% of Medicaid's expenditure is on all care, LTC, and acute services, of beneficiaries (7%) that use LTC services[6]. This no doubt warrants refocusing reform efforts, not just on the LTC but all healthcare delivery needs of these individuals, many seniors, more so urgent considering the imminent increase in the numbers of seniors that would likely need these services in the coming years. Here again, the efforts of any reforms would be toward achieving the DHDO, against the backdrop of the most basic economic principles of the proper allocation and use of scarce healthcare delivery resources. Adherence to these principles requires the identification of these resources and projections of the need for them and other resources in the years ahead. With regard the overall healthcare needs of seniors for example, in the U.S., exploring the prevalence and distribution patterns of primary care physicians, of reform of tort laws in relation to the hindrance of malpractice suits to healthcare delivery, and of adequate physician reimbursement, among others would be necessary. So would the adjustments the health insurance industry would need to make in relation to ensuring the changes made to these issues consequent upon thorough process cycle analyses, including the mechanisms identified, for example the healthcare information and communication technologies as required to improve relevant processes, work. With regard the shortage of primary care physicians for example, it might be necessary to deploy these technologies in a variety of ways that would help with ambulatory and domiciliary care, health insurance firms making the necessary adjustments to facilitate reimbursements processing for example under these circumstances. This, to be most efficient and cost-effective might mean insurance firms developing in-house or purchasing the appropriate healthcare ICT. The placement of the healthcare consumer at the center of the healthcare delivery enterprise is gaining currency in most countries, in particular in the developed world, where concepts such as consumer-directed healthcare and patient-centered healthcare have become entrenched healthcare delivery paradigms. These developments have pervasive effects on the health and related industries, such as the health insurance industry, changes they inspire and dictate in the former likely to cascade down the latter. Thus, the need for information by healthcare consumers to assist them make informed decisions on their choice of healthcare providers, even drugs and other treatment, and on matters regarding their health in general, would require the health insurance to make major adjustments to the ways they conduct business. These would include for example, making public data and information hitherto safely in their custody, some of these might include the lists of medical conditions as they change yearly on which their premium pricing strategies in the main rest. In the study on Medicaid mentioned above, Medicaid's LTC users use the program's acute care services much more than non-LTC users, 75% of the spending on LTC, both community-based and institutional care, 25% on acute care and other supportive services[6]. These high-cost recipients represent Medicaid's most disabled and chronically ill, over 50% elderly, one-third, disabled and under age 65, and 11%, adults or children not termed disabled. Should Medicaid not indeed, seek ways to achieve the DHDO, in particular considering the likely increase in the number of these recipients in the years ahead? This is the situation many developed countries confront and would need to address now before their health systems run into serious trouble, financially and otherwise, which would make the need for health insurance firms in these countries instituting the necessary adjustments also necessary. There is no doubt about the high costs of caring for seniors, many with chronic diseases, seeing different doctors, and using a variety of often-costly medications, more so those that are LTC users. Medicaid spends on the average $46,531 on its less than 65 years disabled recipients for the LTC and acute care, $31,112 on the elderly, and $17, 185 on adults, and children[6]. The costs of acute care on elderly LTC users are twice those for non-LTC users, for the disabled seven times those for non-LTC users. Financed by the federal and state governments, Medicaid pays for health and long-term care coverage for over 50 million Americans and supports thousands of healthcare providers in urban and rural areas. It is a major budget item for states, and indeed, for the federal government, and offers opportunities for access to health services, including long-term care for low-income individuals. The Bush administration proposed in January 2003, to cap all federal Medicaid spending, offering some more funds, and the states choice of programs. Even though the National Governors' Association did not agree on it, and in May 2003, Congress acted in keeping with the program's current structure, in place since the establishment of Medicaid in 1965, to increase federal share, streamlining Medicaid expenses would constitute, despite its recent slower spending pace, an inevitable and ongoing goal of the agency. Medicaid is an entitlement program, with government obliged legally to provide benefits to all eligible individuals, which is key issue regarding accessibility or lack of it to the program by many. Besides eligibility issues, which is a crucial point where the private health insurance firms also have a stake in healthcare delivery to these categories of persons. This is because federal contributions, significant portions of the program's funds, would no longer buffer the states, including helping to plug holes literally in Medicare coverage, outpatient prescription drugs and cost-sharing for examples, for roughly 7 million poor seniors and disabled persons enrolled in both Medicare and Medicaid, with the capping of federal matching funds. As with the need for Center for Medicare and Medicaid Services (CMS) to achieve the DHDO, which individuals ineligible for Medicaid, for examples nonelderly or disabled childless adults, who would then have to fund their healthcare including for example, their LTC, would also likely seek to achieve. This would necessitate the private health insurers they engage collaborating in helping them achieve it. This would be more so as these individuals would have the option of healthcare providers, many involved with Medicaid, hence its requirements, including the implementation of the relevant healthcare information and communication technologies to boost service quality and facilitate the achievement of the DHDO, as opposed to those not doing so that health insurance firms might be dealing with. The need for health insurers to be competitive would be the incentive not just for implementing such technologies, among other adjustments, but for their preference engaging healthcare providers who had. The chances of these scenarios occurring are even likelier with states chipping in their own funds to Medicaid, an incentive for them to manage the program and curtail costs. With costs to both federal and state governments since quite high and variable, and states not sure to receive the right matching funds, Medicare spending also on the increase, as is spending on employment-based health insurance, the need to achieve the DHDO is not in doubt. Medicaid reaches a significant proportion of low-income persons and families, helping to decrease the percentage of the country's uninsured and to prevent it increasing. However, differences between states, and they could be significant, in the extent of coverage for persons for which federal matching funds, which increase or decrease with the states' fortunes, theoretically, although often does not so materialize, variations due in part to the availability of employer-sponsored insurance coverage, and policy preferences, that sometimes compromise access to health services to many. The point here is that government-sponsored services do not always provide all the healthcare coverage that individuals need, and that private health insurance would continue to be important even in countries where public funds essentially pay for healthcare, such as the U.K., and Canada. Another crucial point is that even government sponsored insurance programs would need to ensure the delivery of qualitative health services efficiently and cost-effectively lest their finances become problematic, which could interfere with their ability to deliver qualitative services, and indeed to achieve the DHDO. In other words, health insurance in the public or private sector is going to require some fundamental changes to its operations in light of ongoing developments in the health system occasioned by factors health and nonhealth that drive the health system. A crucial aspect of the fundamental changes that the health insurance industry would need to make concerns accountability, and again, we will use Medicaid to exemplify this issue, whose 'abusive financing scheme' in some states, the General Accounting Office (GAO) and the Inspector General of HHS (OIG) had noted. They involved some states drawing down federal Medicaid matching funds without a parallel spending of state-only funds, for examples via mechanisms such as payment adjustments to Disproportionate Share (DSH) hospitals, and payments to local public hospitals and nursing facilities under "upper payment limits" (UPLs). With these schemes states not paying all if any of its matching funds to complement those paid by the federal government, they increase the effective federal matching rate relative to the specified nominal matching rate. These abuses necessitated the statutory caps on federal Medicaid payments Congress slammed in 1991 and 1993 in reaction to the phenomenal increase in federal spending on DSH hospitals. State-specific DSH caps saved the federal government $10.4 billion between 1998 and 2002, and an extra $30 billion over the next five years, regulatory changes on UPLs, over $64 billion in over 10 years[6]. Accountability in the private health insurance sector would also be crucial to the overall efforts to achieve the DHDO, for example, and would require besides institutional regulatory changes the implementation of appropriate healthcare information and communication technologies. These technologies for example would facilitate billing and reimbursements and to ensure their accuracy, including technologies with differential accessibility by patient, provider, and insurer to eliminate or at least reduce the current high rate of disagreements over the accuracy of provider's bills.

The changes that those in the health industry would spawn in the health

insurance industry would be legion. Many of these changes would be in keeping with the industry's requirement for survival, as competition due to those firms willing to make the necessary changes and evolve in parallel with the health industry, even in health jurisdictions funded with public funds as noted earlier, intensifies. When a firm of private GPs announced in the U.K., in 2004 that it planned to make its services available nationwide, and it was obvious that many patients were ready to abandon the country's National Health Service (NHS) and pay for their care in the private sector, questions naturally arose as to why[7]. Some of the patients cited the peace of mind they had going private and being able to reach their doctor anytime, and that it was cheaper than having private medical insurance. The GPs on the other hand were dissatisfied with the level of service they could provide under the NHS. Thus, there were NHS GPs who supplemented their income with private practice, NHS GPs, who did not, and private medical insurance where some GPs that opted out of the NHS completely operated, the competition by insurers private or public for patronage no doubt evident, heightened by the shortage of GPs.. Would these competitors therefore not have to evolve with the changing paradigms of healthcare delivery, for example, with the need to achieve the dual healthcare delivery objectives, at the different levels, personal, health system, and countrywide? Would the NHS not devise means to continue to provide qualitative services despite and pending when it solves its problems of shortage of GPs., for example, investing in telehealth technologies, and other measures to optimize resource allocation and utilization? Does this example not underscore the point that even health insurance in publicly financed health systems would need some adjusting to make in the prevailing healthcare delivery dispensation, and more so in the years ahead? As noted earlier with the shortage of primary care physicians in the U.S., the dearth of GPs in the U.K., whose Department of Health figures showed that it hired 1,535 in 2004 since 1999, still an extra 10,000 GPs needed in 2004, even more now, is a major challenge for the country's NHS. This is more so as also previously noted for the U.S., with the country's population aging, and many retirees expected in a couple of years to put even more pressure on the NHS to provide required services, qualitative, cost-effective and efficient services. Such national health insurance schemes to survive need to ensure a fall in wait lists, and improve access to care besides improving the quality of care delivery other ways, necessary requirements to keep clientele and to justify their existence given the likely continuity of scarcity of medical resources. There is therefore no room for complacency simply because the health system operates on public funds, the taxes and other publicly generated revenues required to fund it unlikely to keep increasing as this has the potential to ruin the country's economy overall. The funds are therefore going to continue to be insufficient to meet the healthcare needs of all, scarcity that should inspire innovative means for resource reallocation and utilization in the most effective and efficient manner, which the widespread implementation of healthcare information and communication technologies would doubtless help achieve. An important aspect of the evolution of healthcare delivery would therefore be the increasing acknowledgement by health jurisdictions of the potential benefits of these technologies to help achieve the DHDO, and on which in realization of this fact, the UK government is investing billions of pounds to improve the NHS. Even way back in 2004, policies introduced aimed at retaining GPs services in the NHS, such encouraging GPs to see patients within two days, establishing the national telephone helpline, NHS Direct, and walk-in-centers in a bid to compete with the private sector. Offering GPs additional funds to keep their surgeries operational in the evenings and at weekends was up for consideration[7]. The significance of healthcare information and communication technologies in the interplay of the health and insurance industries in the future of both is even more evident considering the symbiotic dyadic of progress in healthcare delivery vis-à-vis that in healthcare ICT. The ever-changing knowledge base of the former necessitates the application of new healthcare-ICT driven processes to ensure the continuity of qualitative healthcare delivery, the novel technologies, themselves changing with progress in technological knowledge, emerging technologies thereof stimulating novel healthcare delivery approaches, the process continuing ad infinitum, to ensure ongoing quality assurance. It inconceivable that the health insurance industry would exclude itself from this process upon which it inherently derives much knowledge crucial to determining its operations, for examples premiums pricing, and physician reimbursements. Indeed, several factors somewhat peculiar to the health insurance industry make it obligatory, not least its constant battle with information asymmetry, which unlike in other domains, it 'suffers' rather than its potential clientele, albeit in the main, in taking decisions crucial to its survival. Thus, unlike the doctor's clientele, those of the insurance firm, are the harbingers of information, health information, the firm requires determining critical aspects of the proposed contract between the two, information that the client might not divulge, at least not in full. The industry also gains embracing a process that results in and extols creativity, hence fosters competition, which as Frank H. Knight, one of the founders of the Chicago school of economics, in his *Risk, Uncertainty, and Profit*, eminently observed, perfect competition need not eliminate profits[8]. With, as Knight explained, uncertainty distinct from risk, the probability of an outcome not determinable with the former but determinable with and possible to insure against in the latter, the potential for profits still operating under uncertainty there, the reasons for a firm shunning competition, even if not going to be a 'pack leader' would indeed, be tenuous. Whereas, competition would ferret, the best from the industry's cryptic depths, and as with the healthcare delivery/healthcare information and communication technologies dyadic, create the potential for synergy not just with these domains, but also with others involved in the healthcare delivery enterprise. This could potentially be the wellspring of a similar dynamic feedback mechanism for enduring quality assurance in the industry, as with the mentioned dyadic. Furthermore, the insurance industry, as with every other, is subject to change, inspired from within, or imposed from without, hence has little if any choice than to be adaptive, responding to these changing in ways that would foster not hinder its evolution. Therefore, evolution in the health insurance industry is not just desirable it is unavoidable. In the U.S., Medicaid spending fell by 1.4% in the two thirds of 2006 versus the same period in 2005, the first decline in spending since the program's inception in 1965, as the Bureau of Economic Analysis, noted, a 5.4% decline post-adjustment for the rate of health care inflation[9]. Policies such as moving seniors on the program from nursing homes into the less pricey home health care, improving fraud detection, streamlining the management of high-cost recipients, for example those that have serious chronic diseases, cutting down on payments to healthcare providers were some of the cost-cutting policies adopted by states recently that seem to have worked. Some states even moved certain medication costs to the Medicare prescription drug benefit, which some argue could be the reason for the seeming Medicaid saving, that without the Medicare drug benefit, Medicaid spending would not have changed from the 2005 figures. Let us assume then that were these possibilities plugged there would indeed, be less if any savings, the program, at both states and federal levels would still be seeking ways to curtail its spending, including stepping up the measures mentioned earlier for examples, and introducing new ones. In other words, responding to changes in the coming years that Medicaid would have to due to the anticipated increase in the number of recipients would create additional burden on the program that is still unsure of the best ways to curtail funds even now, yet obliged to. The learning curve of the program would be less steep in the process were it to embrace the need for competition as a fundamental mechanism in conducting its transactions internally and with the various healthcare providers, nursing homes, and the other agencies with which it operates to deliver the services it provides. It would require for example the optimization of resources based on an analysis of the needs, such as the ability to perform the activities of daily living (ADLs) vis-à-vis the cognitive capacities of a senior in determining, among others the needs of that senior in long term care (LTC). Such an analysis, in contradistinction to a wholesale movement of seniors to less expensive home health care, would be more cost saving in the end, costs likely incurred due to the development of new or worsening of existing conditions being in inappropriate facilities or care setting eliminated, not to mention the enhanced quality of life (QOL) of the seniors. Medicaid would also be able, utilizing the appropriate healthcare information and communication technologies, for example, determine the remuneration approaches most suited to healthcare providers. It might perhaps even offering them incentives to implement relevant technologies and broadening their healthcare delivery scope to include service provision, for example, health promotion and wellness services, whose cumulative effects would be the achievement of the dual healthcare delivery objectives (DHDO.) These examples using Medicaid are applicable to programs of similar nature, where public funds provide for insurance coverage for health and related services, and indeed, to private health insurance too. Thus, competition, played out in all domains of healthcare delivery, would be pervasive in the evolution of health insurance in the coming years, again without any likelihood of enforcement by fiat necessary, simply necessitate the potential for even survival, factors and events even alien to the industry would dictate. It would, at least superficially be possible to understand the chagrin of the health insurance firm that confronts its imminent demise that the trade deficit between the US., and other countries seems set to trigger. Yet, in the recent past, the rate of return on U.S. direct investment overseas was just about 1 percentage point over that for all non-financial corporations in the country, for which the higher risks linked with overseas investments, is partly responsible[10]. Furthermore, the rate of return on foreign direct investment in the U.S. is less than that, overall for all domestic non-financial corporations. With foreign competition intensifying in the financial, health insurance industry, better ROI for the foreign competitors, their market share increasing, hence even more profitability accruing to these foreign competitors, despite the typically lower long-term interest rates in key foreign direct investor countries, which could still enable them achieve a positive net return, should the health insurance firm be alarmed? In particular, with the scale economies, access to the extensive U.S. market confers, via sales/distribution affiliates engendering higher return rates in their countries, and in indeed, all returns, offsetting say even low return rates of their U.S. affiliates, could these foreign firms not still have competitive edge over local health insurance firms in the U.S.?

The above is just one possible instance of the externalities dealing with which the health insurance industry would have little choice in the coming years. Even if, in the above scenario, the value of U.S. overseas assets were understated, as some would contend, in the main because of overlooked but potentially substantial exports of intangibles by U.S. direct investors to their overseas affiliates, which would raise the latter's value, that the scenario could increase competitive pressure on the local firms, is not in doubt. There would also be competition between local firms, with which to contend. Thus, competition would be keen in the years ahead, driven not just by developments in the health industry, but also by those outside it, both within and outside a country, developments the health insurance firms, intent on survival and profitability, would unlikely ignore. The results of these developments would likely be just as profound as the measures the firms would need to take to meet their strategic intent. The yardstick for excellence that the firms would need to set would be, besides being industry-based, would have to be individual-based, each firm aiming for goals set from within, tied to corporate strategies, perhaps even higher than industry benchmarks, meeting both of which would stand them in good stead to compete favorably in the emerging dispensation. Health insurance firms would also have to deal with the consequences of the changing market rules in their countries, some of which could have potential implications for their abilities to survive. The concern in some quarters in the U.S., for example of the damage done by the Sarbanes-Oxley Act of 2002 (SOA,) which aims to regulate corporate governance, to the competitiveness of the U.S. capital markets, with businesses going abroad to overseas exchanges and private sources to raise funds, underscores this point[11]. There is no doubt that this Act, passage of which many consider the collapse of Enron and other major corporations in the U.S. corporate world, triggered, could have major effects for the health insurance industry in the country. These effects could directly or indirectly, relate to the competitiveness and profitability of insurance firms, which might need to raise funds in stock exchanges of the home countries of their competitors, for example, hence costs and accessibility to health services by many individuals in the country. Other developments even within the insurance industry, as earlier noted are going to have significant effects on its direction in the years ahead. An example, again from the U.S., is the potential influence of a new study released on November 30, 2006, which indicated Medicare recipients enrolled in private, managed care plans cost the government about $5.2 billion, 12.4% more per enrollee than did those in the fee-for-service program in 2005[12]. The study, released by the Commonwealth Fund, argues for the potential use of these extra funds to close the prescription-drug coverage gap or lowering monthly premiums. Payments to Medicare Advantage plans, which have 5.6 million Medicare beneficiaries, were $922 per recipient more than what the fee-for-service program would have cost, which some consider not a judicious use of scarce resources. Responding to the study, Karen Ignagni, president and CEO of America's Health Insurance Plans, noted that the report exaggerates the payment amounts, AHIP planning to perform its own independent calculations. She further noted that enrollees in the Medical Advantage plans, which Federal law allows to receive higher payments in rural areas and small cities, are happy with the benefits and services that they receive. These findings have no doubt put the future of the Medical Advantage plans in jeopardy, in particular with the recent observation by Rep. Pete Stark, D-Fremont, who will chair the House Ways and Means health subcommittee that private Medicare Advantage plans are overpaid billions of dollars for coverage to seniors that the government could provide less expensively[13]. Indeed, many believe that the Democrats, who take control of Congress in January 2006, would be examining closely what some consider the Bush administration insistence on privatizing Medicare. The outcome of the imminent confrontation, which would certainly involve the health insurance industry, could only be conjectural. As we noted earlier, progress in healthcare delivery and in healthcare information and communication technologies would influence developments in the health insurance industry, an inevitable process a recent poll of 1,389 persons by the Kaiser Family Foundation underscored. The poll found that 71% of individuals in the new 'consumer-directed health plans'

(CDHP)confirmed the argument of this health insurance/healthcare delivery model's proponents that the policies prompted them to consider cost in seeking health services, versus 49% of those with more conventional employer-sponsored coverage[14]. This finding no doubt attests to the fact that the new plans could curtail escalating health-care spending by providing healthcare consumers a financial incentive not only to seek the best healthcare at affordable prices, but also to receive only the care they need. In short, the plans facilitate the achievement of the dual healthcare delivery objectives (DHDO.) Noted Devon Herrick, a health economist at the National Center for Policy Analysis in Dallas, 'It's a cultural shift, when you go to Wal-Mart you don't have to ask about price–it's right there next to the good or service you are buying. Health care is not there yet, but it's getting that way. This is the early stages. We have the incentives to get people more responsible and asking about price.' Nonetheless, the poll also revealed concerns about the plans, with 50% of those enrolled indicating that they would switch plans given a chance, although 55% said the new plans have changed their health services utilization patterns. Many enrollees complained about the dearth of information on which to base their decisions on which healthcare providers to choose among other important decisions that they want to make regarding their healthcare. Over 60% of those in CDHP observed that it is difficult to find high-quality information about the cost of doctors' services and hospital care, and about 50%, that information on quality of care is difficult to find. This, again highlights the key role of healthcare ICT, which could facilitate information dissemination and cost-effectively too, in the evolution of the health insurance industry. The polls also showed concerns about the high deductibles of the plans, sometimes running into hundreds, even thousands of dollars, versus the roughly $20 co-payments healthcare consumers make in the traditional plans, although premiums tend to be higher with the latter, with CDHP clients twice as likely as those in customary plans to go without care due to cost. This no doubt is an undesirable state of affairs. It could limit access to needed care, and from an economic perspective would not augur well for the health insurance industry, or the health system, not to mention the ethico-moral principles violated. This is the more so considering the recent findings revealed in 'The Uninsured and the Affordability of Health Insurance Coverage,' by Lisa Dubay, a research scientist at the Johns Hopkins Bloomberg School of Public Health, and researchers at the Urban Institute published a Nov 30, 2006, The *Health Affairs* Web exclusive[15]. using the 2005 Current Population Survey (CPS) to approximate what percentage of uninsured Americans are eligible for coverage via Medicaid or the State Children's Health Insurance Program (SCHIP), that require financial help to buy health insurance, and could possibly afford insurance, the study found that 25% 56%, and 20%, respectively in each group. Among the uninsured, it found 74% of children eligible for public programs, and 57% and 69% of parents and childless adults, respectively, require help, in other words, a significant proportion of uninsured adults need help buying health insurance. The consequences of these issues for the health system could be dire. For the health insurance industry, a massive movement of clientele for example from the CDHP would mean more costs for example, to those firms in the traditional domain settling healthcare bills, as even the so-called healthier and wealthier that the CDHP seem to attract for now are complaining about costs although about other things as well. It is uncertain that the higher premiums paid in this domain for example would offset the increased costs, in particular as the influx of 'healthier and wealthier' clients could distort adverse selection and the pricing of premiums, albeit for some time. Meantime, the depletion of patronage in the CDHP could threaten the viability of these plans, and the potential of the health system as a whole to achieve the DHDO. The effects of these scenarios would reverberate way beyond the health and insurance industries, with potential adverse consequences for the country's overall economic growth and development. In fact, another recent report of a telephone survey of 2,122 companies conducted in September 2006 sponsored by Kaiser Family Foundation and Health Research and Educational

Trust showed that health insurance costs are increasingly hindering start-up companies and, even preventing would-be entrepreneurs, in particular individuals with pre-existing health issues starting their businesses[16]. The stifling effect of the exorbitant costs of health insurance the survey revealed affect entrepreneurs with businesses less than five years old, who are in the critical stages of building clientele and profits, most devastatingly. Additionally, many start-ups have few workers hence the firms are unable to receive the discounted insurance rates that larger firms do, premiums according to the survey increasing on the average by 8.8% and 7%, for small and large firms, the latter with over 200 employees, respectively.

Considering the key role of small and medium sized enterprises (SMEs) in the overall economy, it is instructive that a 2005 National Association of the Self Employed (NASE) mail survey of over 600 small businesses showed that 51.1% did not, or plan to, offer themselves or their workers, health insurance coverage. One cannot gainsay the potential for these developments to influence the path of the health insurance industry in the years ahead. That 14% of the smallest firms making less than $50,000 yearly offered health insurance, versus 70% of firms making $500,000 or more, according to this survey also is telling, in particular for the inevitable reorientation of policy on health insurance required in dealing with these and other salient issues. Such policy changes would help address the issues raised by such research findings as mentioned above including for example, according to the NASE survey that it costs smaller and larger firms, offering health insurance 18.7% and 2.3% respectively of their gross sales on health coverage. There is no doubt that no economy could afford to kill literally entrepreneurship. Indeed, many states are examining measures to reduce health insurance costs for small businesses, for examples via high-risk pools offering subsidized coverage to persons with current or chronic health problems. In Canada, two major reports released on March 16, 1943, 'Report on Social Security for Canada' and 'Health Insurance Report' by Leonard Marsh and Dr. Heagerty, respectively signaled important defining moments in the history of the country's social security system and health insurance system, respectively. After going through a phase of intense debates and controversies over how much to engage in both, including those in the 1945 Federal Government's Green Book to the Conference on Reconstruction, three welfare programs emerged between 1951 and 1954, namely, Old Age Assistance, Blind Persons' Allowances, and Disabled Persons' Allowances. The Federal Government essentially offered to share at least 50%, 75% for the blind of provincial spending on strictly defined categories of seniors and disabled persons, and passed the means test of income and assets, which helped many, and excluded many. Passage of the Unemployment Assistance Act in 1956, backdated to 1955, helped rectify many of the issues but many years afterward, there was no sharing of many of the expenditures, for example, for healthcare. Half a century later, there have been resolutions of many of the issues involved with the sharing formulae regarding health, federal funding providing roughly up to 35% or more of provincial health care spending. However, new issues for examples regarding access to healthcare to all, and the country spending an increasing percentage of its gross domestic product (GDP) on healthcare, 9.9% in 2004, have surfaced, and would be important, in the future of health insurance in the country. In fact some of these issues are either yet to emerge, or not fully so. An example is that of the effect on the health insurance industry of the anticipated increase in the number of seniors in the country. However, the issue of these seniors retiring creating additional pressure on the country's pension systems seems likely to depend on the response of the citizenry to new laws on retirement such one passed in Ontario for instance to eliminate compulsory retirement in the country with effect from December 12, 2006, such laws likely passed in other provinces such as

Saskatchewan[18]. Would seniors be working longer in the entire country soon? Would there be incentives to do so, or disincentives not to? Would living and working longer, result in a healthier citizenry, in particular would this reduce illness rates and by extension, the rates and types of service utilization by seniors? What would the effects be on health spending of these developments? This last question in particular, coupled with the need for qualitative health services provision in keeping with the guiding principles of the Canada Health Act of 1984, would be crucial to the future of health insurance in the country. As in most Organization for Economic Co-operation and Development (OECD) countries, 73% on the average in 2004, taxes finance most of healthcare costs in Canada, the need for sustainable health systems financing of health systems not in doubt. Nonetheless, the private sector seems set to play an increasing role in healthcare delivery in the country, as private payments for health, including those that private insurance finance and those paid out of the pocket by individuals and their families, the latter significant sources of healthcare financing in countries with low private health insurance levels. Out of pocket health spending for examples range from 51% in Mexico to 37% in Korea of total health spending in 2004, versus an average private health insurance among OECD countries of 6% in the same year. In Canada, private health insurance, an optional, complement to Medicare, constituted 10% to 15% of overall health spending, but would that figure increase in the coming years, in particular with debate on public-private health system in the country intensifying. There is also the Chaillou v. Quebec case, with the Supreme Court in Quebec essentially lifting the ban by the province on provision of health services Medicare covers. With health spending being between 25% and 45% of provincial/territorial budgets, pressure on the public health system is likely to increase with population aging, among other factors threatening to keep health spending high. However, so would that on private health insurance firms. In both cases, the quest to receive qualitative services, in the latter, at reasonable costs, concerning the individual healthcare consumer, would be high, just as it would be with regard governments that to curtail health spending while providing these services. The private health insurance industry would be hard-pressed to ignore these pressures, which would escalate, in particular those from individual healthcare consumers, whose numbers would likely increase as the population ages. In 2004, public coverage of spending on drugs in Canada was 38%. Would this proportion increase or decrease, and would this matter, if the healthcare consumer would have to pay for drugs out of pocket or via private health insurance? What effects would this have on the way private health insurance evolves in Canada? Would the Canadian healthcare consumer not become increasingly discerning, and would this not bounce back on the health insurance industry? The issues and questions we have raised about Canada emphasize the point we made earlier about how the evolution of the health insurance industry worldwide would be inevitably guided by developments in both health and nonhealth domains. The link between pensions issue in the U.K., for example, with that of health and its funding is one clear although complex example. With U.K firms struggling with the cost of providing their employees with pensions, costs on the average to offer a final salary pension scheme, about a fifth of employees' wages, over 40% of salary in some instances. No wonder then that employer groups such as the Confederation of British Industry (CBI) are crying out that high pension costs are harmful to profitability, jobs, and investments. These groups are thus calling on government to act on May's Pensions White Paper to make simpler rules and lessen regulation. While many firms want to meet, pension obligations but are asking employees to make more contributions, as high as 60% in some firms. Even at the risk of contravening the country's age discrimination laws in effect from October 2006, 25% of U.K. firms' pension schemes pay contributions according to age and length of service younger workers thus benefiting from lesser employer pension contributions than older ones[20]. These issues have the potential to affect health in particular in an aging population such as in the U.K, where the government pays the bulk of pensions the funds for which it obtains from taxation, National Insurance contributions, and borrowing. In 2002 the basic state pension paid out to pensioners nearly £38bn. In addition to basic pension, it also funds the Second State Pension (formerly the State Earnings Related Pension System or SERPS), the cost of giving pensioners a minimum income notwithstanding their National Insurance Contributions (the Pension Credit) and housing, council tax and disability benefits, which all totaled nearly £64bn in 2002. This amount would increase based on the country's demography, its seniors population expected to rise in the years ahead. The U.K. government also funds the bulk of health services. With the private sector reeling under the strain of pensions payments, what consequences could this have for economic productivity, and if it could compromise employment, who bears the burden but government? Could this not create additional financial burden on government and its ability to fund the National Health Service (NHS), the increasing spending on which already is of major concern? Would this not change the dynamics of private versus public health insurance, which latter some already construe government as essentially privatizing? The likely increasing involvement of private health insurance in the U.K. health system would mean heightened competition among insurance firms, including local and foreign firms, the influx of which latter would be inevitable. That firms base pension schemes on age and length of service means fewer benefits to younger and early retirees, who would also depend more on government health services and for longer periods, creating additional financial burden on these services. This is not to mention the adverse consequences for the health of many of being unemployed, which the increasing crunch on firms due to higher pension costs could engender. The potential accentuation of these issues by the projected increase in the proportion aged over 65, which the Pensions Commission noted would be by 78% between 2006 and 2050, coupled with the fact that about 15 million individuals of working age are not making any pension provision for their retirement is ominous[21]. This is because the dependence on the state for an income by so many and for health services simultaneously would be immense and strenuous, although studies such as that conducted by the Institute of Fiscal Studies paint a slightly rosier picture. This latter study for example, of persons in their 50s or early 60s, yet to retire suggested these groups would spend on their retirement close to 50% of their wealth accruable from property owned and money inherited. This would if things turned out to be so, also influence the dynamics of the private and public health insurance in the U.K., with resources available for such persons to spare on for example, additional health insurance purchased from the private sector. The state pensions in some other European countries are somewhat higher than in the U.K., although the problems on over-reliance on government largesse remain just as potent in many of them. The average pensioner in Sweden, Holland, France, and Spain receives roughly 70% of their working income, versus the 37% that U.K's basic and second state pensions provide[21]. However, in the U.K., about 18 million people of working age contribute to private pension plans, run by employers and those by self-employed persons, or have partners who do, these schemes paying out in 2002, almost £18bn to their pensioners. Many of the newer schemes base their final payout on the accumulated investment return unrelated to salary or length of service at least not directly, making pensions' funding additionally precarious where the investments of employee and employer contributions in shares, property, and bonds yield no tangible returns for example, with potential consequences for health and health insurance. Pensions costs are also increasing in the public sector, and financed by tax, among others, could create enormous tax burden on future generations, in particular the increased funds the aging population would require. As noted earlier, there are plans in many developed countries to increase the retirement age, as part of the solutions to these problems. This would require convincing not just individuals to work longer, but workers to create employment opportunities for older persons, and an environment conducive for those still at work to operate, to encourage them to stay on their jobs longer. For example, this could involve the deployment of the appropriate information technologies to enhance their visual and auditory acumen, even to encourage them to exercise while at work, and in general, to improve their health and well-being, all of which, again, have potential implications for the health insurance industry. The above discussion clearly shows the interplay of a variety of factors both health and nonhealth in the future of the health insurance industry in different countries. The industry would no doubt have to pay attention to developments in these different domains, including in the healthcare information and communication technologies domain, and adapt appropriately to changes that could determine success or otherwise in the industry. These adaptations, would also feed into developments in health and indeed, all these other domains, somehow modifying them, the interactions between the health insurance and these other industries therefore potentially mutually beneficial.

References

1. Congressional Budget Office, "The Budget and Economic Outlook: Fiscal Years 2005 to 2015," January 2005, p.3.

2. Available at: http://news.bbc.co.uk/2/hi/health/3484706.stm Accessed on November 26, 2006

3. Available at: http://healthaffairs.org/blog/2006/11/17/insurance-deconstructing-insurance/#more-89 Accessed on November 26, 2006

4. Edwards, Chris. *Downsizing the Federal Government*. CATO Institute, Washington. D.D. p. 3

5. Available at:
http://www.macleans.ca/topstories/national/article.jsp?article=2006_11_24_11 64400791 Accessed on November 26, 2006

6. Available at: http://www.kff.org/medicaid/7576.cfm Accessed on November 26, 2006

7. Available at: http://news.bbc.co.uk/2/hi/health/3571737.stm Accessed on November 26, 2006

8. Knight, Frank H. (1885-1972) Title: *Risk, Uncertainty, and Profit* Published: Boston, MA: Hart, Schaffner & Marx; Houghton Mifflin Company, 1921

9. Available at:

http://www.kaisernetwork.org/daily_reports/print_report.cfm?DR_ID=41256
&dr_cat=3 Accessed on November 30, 2006.

10. Available at: http://bea.gov/bea/papers/darkmatter_10_2006.pdf Accessed
on November 30, 2006.

11. Available at: http://www.cato.org/pub_display.php?pub_id=6624 Accessed
December 1, 2006

12. B. Biles, L. Hersch Nicholas, B. S. Cooper, E. Adrion, and S. Guterman, The
Cost of Privatization: Extra Payments to Medicare Advantage Plans — Updated
and Revised, The Commonwealth Fund, November 2006 Available at:
http://www.cmwf.org/publications/publications_show.htm?doc_id=428546
Accessed on December 1, 2006

13. Available at: http://www.sfgate.com/cgi-
bin/article.cgi?f=/c/a/2006/12/01/MNG33MN8O51.DTL&hw=medicare+adva
ntage&sn=001&sc=1000
Accessed on December 1, 2006

14. Available at: http://www.washingtonpost.com/wp-
dyn/content/article/2006/11/29/AR2006112901384_pf.html Accessed on
December 1, 2006

15. Available at:
http://www.kaisernetwork.org/daily_reports/rep_index.cfm?DR_ID=41359
Accessed on December 1, 2006

16. Available at:

http://www.kaisernetwork.org/daily_reports/rep_index.cfm?DR_ID=41353

Accessed on December 1, 2006

17. Available at: http://www.oecd.org/dataoecd/19/13/36956887.pdf

Accessed on December 1, 2006

18. Available at: http://www.labour.gov.on.ca/english/news/2006/06-120.html

Accessed on December 1, 2006

19. Available at:

http://www.oecd.org/document/37/0,2340,en_2649_37407_36986213_1_1_1_37

407,00.html Accessed on December 1, 2006

20. Available at: http://news.bbc.co.uk/go/pr/fr/-/2/hi/business/5186780.stm

Accessed on December 2, 2006

21. Available at: http://news.bbc.co.uk/2/hi/business/4378366.stm Accessed

on December 2, 2006

Healthcare Agenda Anew

The 35 million perennially unemployed a.k.a, working poor in the U.S.,
persons whose income is less than 200% of the federal poverty level, who have
little, if any skills, yet constitute an attractive labor option for employers in
particular in the healthcare, hospitality, retail, and manufacturing industries,
sizeable turnover costs notwithstanding, are attracting a different kind of
attention lately. With pressure to swap the 7.5 million illegal immigrant workers
in the country with homegrown workers mounting, the political and economic
dimensions of these issues are increasingly under scrutiny, but is the health
dimension receiving such attention, or enough of it, and should it not? The
country's total spending makes up 15.3% of its GDP in 2004, the highest
percentage among Organization for Economic Cooperation and Development
(OECD) countries whose average the same year was 8.9%[1]. That year,
Switzerland, Germany, and France spent 11.6%, 10.9%, and 10.5% of their GDP,

respectively on health. In total health spending per capita terms, the U.S. spent US$6,100, adjusted for purchasing power parity, on health, over twice the US$2,550 OECD average in the same year, health spending per capita in the country between 1999 and 2004, up in real terms by an average of 5.9% per annum, versus the OECD average of 5.2% per annum[1]. Are these figures for the U.S., likely to increase or decrease? What role is population aging going to play in this regard? Would the health dimensions of the immigrant/working poor issue also play a significant role? Life expectancy has increased in many OECD countries over the past four decades, 77.5 years in 2003/4 in the U.S., where it increased by 7.6 years between 1960 and 2003, in Japan and Canada by more than 14 years and by 8.6 years, respectively[1]. Many of the seventy six million baby-boomers born in the U.S., between 1946 and 1964 would be retiring in the next five years, with potential adverse consequences for the labor market, the need for workers with the knowledge and skills many of these individuals have likely to escalate, in particular with regard certain occupations, including in the health industry. We should note though that there is a major rethink of the idea of mandatory retirement in many developed countries, including Canada, where a law would be effective December 12, 2006 in Ontario eliminating mandatory retirement, for example, other provinces such as Saskatchewan likely to follow suit[2]. Yet, the consequences of the retirement of baby boomers for healthcare delivery, and indeed, for the economies of developed countries are still potentially profound. In spite of the comparatively high level of health spending in the U.S., for example, the country has fewer physicians per capita than most other OECD countries, 2.4 practicing physicians per 1 000 population, less than the OECD average of 3.0 in 2004[3]. What is more, the country's pool of first-line doctors, primary care physicians, is fast drying up, with fewer younger doctors keen to replace retiring GPs[4]. With large numbers of baby boomers likely to need increasing medical attention, is a crisis looming, hollering for health agenda anew? There is no doubt that lack of access to needed healthcare could only increase morbidities and mortalities, the excess and in the main avoidable burden of disease in both health and economic terms, likely to increase the budgetary pressure under which the country's health services currently reel. The shortage of healthcare personnel is not peculiar to the U.S., or restricted to primary care doctors. The U.S., had 7.9 nurses per 1 000 population in 2002, fewer than the OECD average of 8.3., and in terms of acute care hospital beds, which many of these seniors would increasingly need, the U.S., had 2.8 per 1 000 population in 2004, versus the OECD average of 4.1 beds per 1 000 population that same year. With regard acute hospital care beds, many OECD countries have made efforts to reduce hospital admission rates and stays including increasing the number of day surgeries over the past two decades, the number of hospital beds per capita down from 4.4 beds per 1 000 population in 1980 to 2.8 in 2004[1]. This issue also raises important questions about the future of hospitals that tie tightly with those of the delivery of qualitative health services simultaneously reducing health spending, in other words, the achievement of the dual healthcare delivery objectives (DHDO,) highlighting the need for attention to a significant source of soaring health spending, those on hospitalizations and related costs. Thus, would it be necessary, or appropriate to continue to reduce the number of hospital beds per capita, and what would be the consequences of this for health services delivery in particular to seniors, and others, including the millions of working poor and illegal immigrants mentioned above, and should these issues not be major aspects of the new healthcare agenda? The fact is that serious considerations of such issues would reveal the complicated cross-agenda on which contemporary health policy review predicates. That considerations of alternative healthcare delivery models for seniors for example that would reduce their current and likely more intense future hospital utilization, with major costs implications, would lead to those of the widespread implementation of appropriate healthcare information and communication technologies (ICT), that could facilitate ambulatory and domiciliary care, and the achievement of the

DHDO is doubtless. These considerations might also result in increased focus on the potential benefits of these technologies, and indeed, other solutions, in organizing and actualizing innovative health services to meet the needs of different segments of society, including the working poor and illegal immigrants, among the necessary package of multidimensional approaches to addressing issues regarding who, any country could ill-afford to ignore. Consider the issue of diabetes, whose prevalence has increased in recent decades in many countries, including the U.S., where for example obesity rate among adults, was 30.6% in 2002, the highest among OECD countries. The rate in Mexico in 2000 was 24.2%, and in 2004, in the United Kingdom and Canada, 23.0%, 22.4%, respectively[3]. With the established link between obesity and chronic diseases such as diabetes, asthma, and cardiovascular diseases, is the increasing obesity rate in the U.S., indeed, among both the rich and poor, coupled with the increased prevalence of diabetes for example, among certain racial groups, not likely to increase the prevalence of these conditions, with increased healthcare costs, hence health spending? With 16 million Americans, 5.9% of the total population, diagnosed with diabetes by 1999, the number increasing, African Americans, Hispanics, American Indians, and Japanese Americans, Chinese Americans, Filipino Americans, and Korean Americans, all at increased risk of developing diabetes[5], would any serious efforts to ensure the achievement of the DHDO not involve ensuring required healthcare delivery to its different peoples? Should this issue also not be on the list of the new health agenda? Clearly, the need for such agenda is urgent in the U.S., and many other countries, with the increase in health spending that in many cases is disproportionate to the rate of spending rise in other sectors of their economy, and is evidently unsustainable. With healthcare delivery an assemblage of complicated transactions between a variety of disparate entities at different levels of different sectoral domains both health and nonhealth related, the potential issues for considerations in any effort not just to improve health services delivery but also to seek to achieve the DHDO are legion. This warrants a systematic approach to these issues that would involve in particular health jurisdictions, decomposition/exposition exercises that would reveal the general and peculiar issues requiring focus, and inclusion in a comprehensive health agenda under the observation/issue decomposed, and indeed, the potential solutions to them. These process cycle analyses for example would, by exposing the interlocking processes involved in a particular transaction that constitutes a component of the many that result in an aspect of the overall healthcare delivery enterprise, reveal mechanisms by which we could make it more efficient and cost-effective. These mechanisms might include the implementation of particular healthcare ICT, whose prospects of leading to the achievement of the DHDO, would in turn inform the need to consider the potential role of these technologies in healthcare delivery a major healthcare agenda issue. Considering the chances of the enduring dyadic of progress of knowledge in healthcare delivery and in these technologies to spawn creativity and innovation in both that would feed into either, creating a synergy-cum-driver for the required ongoing quality assurance essential for perpetuating the gains of the DHDO, a new orientation to healthcare policy formulation and implementation is ripe. Indeed, it is imperative for any health system, were it to meet the stringent requirements for success, let alone survival in the new healthcare delivery dispensation, wherein the healthcare consumer is at the center-stage so to say, of the healthcare delivery enterprise.

With the healthcare consumer's expectations of health services delivery increasingly sophisticated, the increasing availability of health information, in particular via the Internet, etching away at the crusty pervasive information asymmetry that hitherto compromised the empowerment of healthcare consumers in matters relating to their health, the burgeoning options and the enhance ability to discern among which result, are instructive. This is so because of the immense implications of these developments among others for future healthcare delivery, and indeed, for the ability of health systems to survive, as the need to justify their existence increasingly coincides with that to satisfy their clientele. This would be the case regardless of the funding model of the health system, as healthcare consumer behavior has similar core origins, the need to be alive and to be healthy, critical among them. As far as there are options therefore, even if untested and proofs if any of their claims of efficacy lack the methodological rigor of Western science, peoples would seek alternative means of achieving these twin goals. In countries such as Canada, with public funds the main source of payments for health services provision, health jurisdictions would still need therefore, to operate within the basic principles of economics. Thus, they would need to operate under budgetary constraints as resources are, and would always be scarce, as long as the country, and for that matter, any country could not satisfy all of everyone's needs. They would also need to determine and adopt the best means to allocate and utilize scarce healthcare resources efficiently and cost-effectively, as competition, even among health jurisdictions play out more dramatically in the coming years, not to mention, between public and private health services. In Quebec only, at least for now, the Supreme Court has ruled that individuals could seek health services in the private sector, even for conditions Medicare covers, and several other provinces are openly in favor of a parallel private health system. It seems conceivable that health jurisdictions even across provinces and territories would for competitive reasons, establish and others discontinue services that are more or less cost-effectively and efficiently delivered, respectively, a process that could result in closures of unviable, economically, and otherwise, clinical units, service programs if not whole hospitals. These measures are in fact happening, as the progressive decline in hospital beds among OECD countries, including Canada, mentioned earlier shows, although perhaps not as intensively as in the past few decades, the increasing empowerment of the healthcare consumer likely to accelerate their occurrence in the years ahead. It seems paradoxical that persons receiving healthcare that public funds maintain would make it moribund. Nonetheless, this is the emerging reality of contemporary healthcare delivery that calls for new healthcare agenda in all countries including Canada, as the more individuals seek required services they lacked or could not readily access in their health jurisdiction, in another health jurisdiction, the higher the loss of patronage in the former. This could eventually compromise the ability of the health jurisdiction depleted of patronage to justify the continued existence of certain services, or for that matter, its very own. This underscores the need for health jurisdiction even in countries where taxes and other revenues generated from the public fund health services not to discountenance the concept of the DHDO, the achievement of which the widespread implementation and utilization of the relevant healthcare ICT could facilitate. Even where these technologies necessitate service rationalization, for example, the need for as many hospital beds as before, they would spawn services that are more efficient and cost-effective than previously, which are the goals every health jurisdiction would need to achieve to survive, yet be able to meet, and indeed, surpass its healthcare delivery mandates. The rationalization of services that would ensue in the example given above, such as the increased use of ambulatory and home patient care delivery/monitoring technologies, would help reduce the adverse effects of the shortage of primary care physicians mentioned above, which Canada also, and indeed other countries such as the U.K have. This is besides other measures, for example, utilizing the doctors available more in clinical rather than administrative positions, a role diffusion that only aggravates an already difficult situation. Canada spends more than many OECD in terms of total health spending per capita, US$3165 in 2004 (adjusted for purchasing power parity), versus the OECD average of US$2550, although much lower than those of countries such as the U.S., which in the same year spent US$6100 per capita, and those of Switzerland and Norway[6]. Many argue that the country could not afford to keep spending increasing proportions of its wealth on healthcare delivery, but even if it could, could it not deliver the same and even higher quality health services to its peoples for less money, and if it could why should it not do so? The same questions apply to the U.K., Australia, New Zealand, and indeed, many other countries with varying mixtures of private and public health services, as private payments for health services also exist in Canada, although only for services Medicare does not fund. Why should these and indeed, any other country not speed up efforts to promote the widespread implementation and utilization of healthcare ICT for example at every health jurisdictional level, technologies that researches have shown could help achieve the dual healthcare delivery objectives? The point here is that controlling increasing healthcare costs would be a major issue in the coming years in many countries, hence would feature prominently in the new healthcare agenda. A Rand Corp. study published in the September/October 2005 issue of the journal *Health Affairs*, for example, showed that the widespread implementation and effective use of electronic medical record (EMR) systems and other healthcare ICT could save the U.S., US$162 billion a year[7]. It also showed that computerized physician order entry (CPOE) systems could eradicate two million adverse drug events (ADEs) in the ambulatory setting and 200,000 in hospitals, the implications for the reduction of apparently preventable but cost-provoking morbidities, hence that of health spending, clear. Yet, another study, Agency for Healthcare Research and Quality (AHRQ)-funded, and collaboration between the Medical Group Management Association (MGMA) and the Minnesota School of Public Health published in the same issue of *Health* indicated a slow rate of automating among healthcare providers in the U.S., particular among the smaller practices. It found that just 12.5% of practices with fewer than 5 physicians using EMR versus 19.5% for those with twenty or more doctors for example, and 14.1% of all practices[7]. In fact, the results of the Commonwealth Fund 2006 International Health Policy

Survey showed that the U.S and Canada are way behind other industrialized countries in healthcare ICT implementation[8]. The survey in which more than 6,000 primary care doctors in Australia, Canada, Germany, the Netherlands, New Zealand, the U.K, and the U.S participated showed that primary care physicians in the U.S. lack the tools or support to provide the best care possible to patients, which translates to not achieving the DHDO. This is ominous for frontline services delivery in particular as earlier noted, with the imminent surge in the population of seniors who need these services most. Should these issues not in fact top the new healthcare agenda in the U.S, not just because of the ethico-moral obligation it has to provide its citizens qualitative health services, but also because it makes intuitive sense to pursue the DHDO, and to avoid doing otherwise whose adverse consequences for its overall health and economic growth are potentially devastating? Should the country not be addressing the problems hindering the adoption of these technologies who lack, among other reasons make a chore for its primary care doctors to function at the comparatively higher levels of their counterparts in other industrialized countries, or practice without basic decision support systems (DSS) that could improve health outcomes and curtail health spending? Why for example, as the study showed, and despite the enormous amounts the country spends of healthcare, should U.S. primary care doctors be less likely than those in many of these other developed countries not be able to offer the healthcare consumer access to healthcare outside office hours? Why should they lack the healthcare ICT to alert them to potentially harmful drug interactions? Should part of the agenda not be what to do to encourage these and other healthcare providers, and indeed, healthcare consumers and other healthcare stakeholders to acquire, implement and use the relevant healthcare ICT that would facilitate the achievement of the DHDO at each stakeholder level? Would this not make it likelier for doctors in the U.S., not to think for example that implementing these technologies only benefit health plans? Do healthcare ICT vendors not have a stake in the widespread implementation of these technologies, and need they not engage in the concerted efforts to promote their widespread adoption, and is it not possible for health plans to also embark on this healthcare ICT-adoption drive? The survey mentioned above showed that 40% or more of U.S. and Canadian primary care physicians admitted difficulty identifying patients overdue for a test or preventive care, versus 19% or less in the other countries studied. It also indicated that fewer than one of five U.S. and Canadian primary care doctors have access to healthcare ICT, which an enabling milieu for ensuring high-quality patient care, the U.K., distinct, among these countries in having healthcare information and communication technologies systems to track medical errors. Seventy nine percent of its primary care doctors noted they were able to document all Ads, versus between 7% and 41% in other countries, 37% in the U.S.

Clearly, the role of these technologies in the future of healthcare delivery is

not in doubt, as are not, the benefits to a country's health system, and indeed, to its economic growth and sustainable development of achieving the dual healthcare delivery objectives as the example of Switzerland illustrates.

A recent OECD/World Health Organization (WHO) report showed that Switzerland's health system meets the crucial objectives of good health outcomes and universal health coverage, but at a high financial cost[9]. The new report noted that only the U.S., among OECD countries surpasses Switzerland regarding health spending as a percentage of GDP, yet other OECD countries perform equally well, or even better, at lower cost, which underscores the point we made earlier about embracing the concept of the DHDO. Switzerland spent 11.5% of its GDP on health in 2003, versus the 8.8% OECD average, its health spending increasing progressively, between 1994 and 2004, by 2.4%, versus the 1.5% OECD average. The report, expressed concerns about a potential escalation in health spending due to the country's aging population, which it has in common with other developed countries, among other factors, which would unlikely be sustainable, and recommended the country came up with more cost-effective policies to gain better control of future health outlay. Measures suggested include as Dr. Marc Danzon, WHO's Regional Director for Europe observed 'Investing in prevention and health promotion programs would help Swiss health authorities focus on important public health issues such as tobacco and alcohol consumption and on areas in need of more attention such as mental health and obesity. This would promote health and prevent disease in the whole population, by actively targeting people at high risk.' Despite its high spending Switzerland, spends just 2.2% of this on disease prevention and health promotion versus the 2.7% OECD average[9]. The report also recommended that the country revisited its physician remuneration systems, to provide strong incentives to increase efficiency and cost-effectiveness, and its health insurance system, limiting the possibilities of insurers selecting patients based on their health risk, and ensuring insurers select healthcare providers based on quality. It also recommended that the healthcare consumer able to choose the best insurance coverage for the least premium, and that competition regarding insurance and health services provision should cross canton boundaries, these recommendations highlighting some of the points we made earlier, the key role that healthcare information and communications technologies would play in actualizing them equally clear. They also attest to the need for Canada and the U.S., for examples, and indeed, other countries to take the necessary measures to encourage the acquisition and use of these technologies by their doctors and other healthcare professionals. There is no doubt regarding the recognition of the benefits of these technologies in these two countries, both of which continue to spend millions of dollars on healthcare ICT, and in many others where they still do not feature as prominently as they should in the healthcare delivery process. The slow pace of their adoption by healthcare professionals attests to the need for the matter to be high on the new healthcare agenda in both countries considering the potential of these technologies to help in achieving the DHDO. This would enable the in-depth exploration of the various issues involved in accelerating the pace of the universal adoption of the technologies. Cost no doubt is a major issue preventing the widespread adoption of these technologies by doctors, particularly those in smaller practices, although there are many others, including technophobia, and concern about the technologies compromising productivity by slowing down doctors' routine operations both during the transition from paper-based to digital processes, and thereafter. Yet other doctor worry about returns on investment (ROI), the sometimes-steep learning curves for both the doctors and their staff required to use the technologies successfully, interoperability with legacy and disparate systems, and maintenance and other costs, relating to total costs of ownership (TCO) of the technologies. With the substantial investments of these two and indeed many other developed countries in healthcare ICT, in particular with regard establishing nationwide electronic health networks, they cannot afford to let these investments essentially come to naught with the complementary EMR that doctors, and other healthcare providers need to hook up with these networks lacking. It is therefore in their best interests and those of all stakeholders at that to be active regarding the promotion of the widespread adoption of these technologies. One cannot over-emphasize the intricate interrelationships of healthcare delivery, healthcare information and communication technologies, and the overall economic growth and development of a country, which is another compelling reason for countries and health systems to embrace these technologies in the new healthcare delivery dispensation, hence for the matter to be high on their new health agenda. The

Canadian economy for example is remarkable, output and employment growth even more, unemployment rate least since 1974, inflation in check, and general government/current account balances, in surplus[10]. The standard of living of Canadians is one of the highest among OECD countries, yet, in the past few years except in 2005, business sector hourly productivity growth has not been that high. There is no doubt about the need for the country to increase productivity growth and for its fiscal and social policies to be sustainable, in particular with the imminent increase in seniors likely to retire, with the potential to reduce the country's labor force. There is also the additional increased pressure on the health system with the chances of further escalation in health spending. These issues, mandate focus, among others, on ways to reduce health spending while not compromising healthcare delivery, but in fact improving it, considering the significant role a healthy populace would likely play in increasing the country's economic productivity. As evident from our discussion thus far, healthcare delivery is an important aspect of both the lives of the citizenry of a country, and indeed, of its economy, the association between health and the economy imbued with intrinsic bidirectional causality on the one hand, driven by an imperative predicated on exigencies and ongoing evolutionary forces, both health and nonhealth. This underscores the need for all sectors of the economy to participate in the efforts to secure the widespread adoption of healthcare ICT for example, and there are indeed, notable examples of such efforts, as the recent gift of C$2.5 million by TELUS, a Telco, to the Alberta Children's Hospital Foundation shows. The gift is to support commitment to providing high quality healthcare services to Albertans. The Foundation used the gift to buy the Vocera Communications System, a sophisticated hands-free, voice-controlled communications device, which enables child healthcare providers at the hospital to communicate and share information utilizing a high-tech badge. The hospital is the first in the country to use this technology, expected to improve the efficiency and cost-effectiveness of service delivery, and patient safety. Certainly, this sort of gesture from the private sector would help significantly in the pervasive deployment of healthcare ICT in the country, hence needs encouraging[11]. Indeed, not only should countries have a healthcare information and communication technologies policy, this policy should incorporate the expected roles of various economic sectors distinctly and encourage each to work on and deliver on them. This policy would also need to address the multiple technical, legal, and other issues that surround the widespread implementation of these technologies, and because these issues are not static, the policy would require periodic updating to keep pace with changes that could profoundly influence its implementation in different domains. The policy would need to stipulate the nature and extent of the involvement of organs of state, for example, federal and state/provincial governments in the development of healthcare information and communication technologies standards for example, which many believe they should not all meddle with in the first place. There seems to be a consensus on this matter in the U.S., at least that government should simply promote the facilitation of these standards and support those developing them. An example of the latter would be SureScripts, the country's largest provider of electronic prescribing services, which in mid-November 2006 announced that it had developed a new certification status. The company stated that this certification status would recognize physician software products/service vendors and others, who develop more functionality. This would be to encourage efforts at improving electronic prescribing, and healthcare interoperability in the U.S[12]. According to the firm, to qualify for the GoldRx status, vendors need to train their installed base on new pharmacy capabilities, include pharmacy interoperability in their standard implementation repertoire, devote the appropriate resources to interoperability, and see workflow progress as more than just electronic prescribing. This means that they need to incorporate in their software systems medication history, formulary, and eligibility information for examples. The GoldRx certification status complements existing standards in the U.S., for examples the Healthcare Information Technology Standards Panel (HITSP), developed to define technical standards, and the Certification Commission for Healthcare Information Technology (CCHIT), to certify vendors in compliance of HITSP standards. SureScripts intends to announce its first round of GoldRx recipients on February 27, 2007. This example again, highlights the need for inter-sectoral collaboration at various levels, and that of the new health agenda to promote it as does the plan by five major employers in the U.S., to offer their employees access to personal health records (PHR) technology. This essentially gives the workers their very own electronic medical record (EMR), they could use however they choose, whenever[13]. This plan would give nearly 2.5 million workers and their dependents access to their PHR via any computer. An independent nonprofit body would put the records together the information stored in a database, to which employees would be able to access the database and to choose who else has access, for example, their doctors, and other healthcare providers. Applied Materials, BP America, Inc., Intel Corp., Pitney Bowes, and Wal-Mart are the firms involved with this plan, which they envisaged by eliminating paperwork would slash administrative and transactions costs, reduce care duplication, and medical errors, hence improve patient safety.

Any attempt to recruit healthcare information and communication technologies in helping achieve the dual healthcare delivery objectives essentially includes facilitating access to and expanding access to health coverage, both of which therefore need to feature equally prominently in the new healthcare agenda. These technologies could no doubt help many hitherto excluded persons gain access to needed healthcare, for example, those living in remote and rural, underserved areas. Incidentally, many of these individuals contribute significantly to their countries' economy hence it is in the overall interests of these countries for them to be healthy and strong. In any case, why should a segment of a country's population not have access to healthcare services? There are clearly other issues besides economics involved in the improvement of access to health services by all. There is always a compelling reason for an individual to be healthy, which is in fact personal to that person, although not necessarily obvious, or not potentially ignored by that individual, for a variety of other reasons. Even the physical presence of a severely disabled person could give succor to both the individual and the relatives, which could make a significant difference to the quality of life (QOL) of both. In other words, being alive is our natural state, and the tendency to die a by-product of this natural state that is and would probably be eventually controllable by each person. Thus, we could argue that our tendency to stay alive is essentially a competitive process between those forces internal and external tending to expire us. It is also likely for the forces that keep us alive to overcome those that threaten to kill us as we not only understand these competitive forces better, but also gain more control over them. At the very least for now, we should prevent external forces such as lack of access to health services sending people prematurely to their graves. Not even the contention of some that we are going to become frail and incur avoidable costs on society would be valid, and that is not to say that they are even now, when for example, appreciate the implications of a variety of research findings by scientists. One for example, over half a century ago that animals compelled to survive on 30% to 30% less calories than their normal amount had resistance to many age-related diseases, such as diabetes, cancer and heart disease, and lived a lot longer is instructive, although with the increasing prevalence of obesity, not one lesson we imbibed. It is also likely that the more we know what to do to prevent the cells mitochondria 'poisoning' our DNA and other genetic materials and indeed, other cellular components with the by-products of its biochemical metabolic processes, in particular the oxidants, the less would the be pace and effect of aging, and the loner and healthier we would live. In fact, scientists discovered over a decade ago that the addition of an extra copy of a gene referred to as Sir2 resulted in yeast cells living 30% longer, scientists presently attributing the advantages of calorie restriction for health and indeed, the repair of our genetic materials to Sir2 or other sirtuin genes. Could there be anything adverse in society having citizens living longer, but also healthier, able to contribute meaningfully to its progress? Should this not be in fact what developed countries in particular those which not only have an aging population, but not enough younger peoples to replace these seniors when they expire? Should such countries, in addition to ensuring access to qualitative health services, cost-effectively to all, including seniors, not be investing significantly in research that would help elucidate the aging mechanisms with a view to enabling us to understand and have more control over these processes? Healthcare delivery to seniors and indeed, to all those lacking access to health services cannot wait until we find the solution to aging, though, which is why access to care by all should be prominent on the new health agenda. Individuals not only should receive the required qualitative healthcare, they should within a reasonable time period, both of which issues still plague health systems in developed countries whose health systems are far more advanced than those in developing countries. It is again, the case that the widespread deployment of healthcare information and communication technologies could help ease these two problems, wait times in particular, in itself, deserving of major policy attention, as many patients' illnesses worsen while they wait for say, surgery, some even dying before they had a chance to see the surgeon. The point here is that every health system would need to pay more attention to the variety of issues germane to it, and that would ensure that it delivers qualitative health services cost-effectively and efficiently, in effect, achieving the dual healthcare delivery objectives. The new healthcare delivery dispensation is going to be ever more complex that failure to pay attention to and devise appropriate policies to address them would spell doom, inevitably for the health jurisdiction. This again is so, considering the many forces both internal and external at play, essentially with a tendency to enjoin the basic principles of economics, even in public funded health jurisdictions. These principles would become the guiding light of health services delivery in the future, made more potent by, albeit even if it spawned accountability itself, predicated on the need to survive. In short, health systems of the future would be self-healing, out of necessity, than compulsion. This general tendency would have far-reaching consequences for the way we perceive and conduct our affairs in not just health but also in other domains of our lives.

References

1. Available at: www.oecd.org/health/healthdata Accessed on December 3, 2006

2. Available at: http://www.labour.gov.on.ca/english/index.html Accessed on December 3, 2006

3. Available at:
http://www.oecd.org/country/0,3021,en_33873108_33873886_1_1_1_1_1,00.htm
l Accessed on December 3, 2006

4. Garibaldi RA, Popkave C, Bylsma W. Career plans for trainees in internal medicine residency programs. Acad Med. 2005; 80:507-512.

5. Carter JS, Pugh JA, Monterrosa A. Non-insulin-dependent diabetes mellitus in minorities in the United States. *Ann Intern Med* 1996; 125(3):221-32. (AHRQ Grant HS07397).

6. Available at:
http://www.oecd.org/country/0,3021,en_33873108_33873277_1_1_1_1_1,00.htm
l# Accessed on December 3, 2006

7. Available at: http://www.healthcareitnews.com/story.cms?id=3653 Accessed on December 3, 2006

8. Available at:

http://www.cmwf.org/newsroom/newsroom_show.htm?doc_id=419135
Accessed on December 3, 2006

9. Available at:

http://www.oecd.org/document/47/0,2340,en_33873108_33873838_37562223_1
_1_1_1,00.html Accessed on December 3, 2006

10. Available at:

http://www.oecd.org/document/29/0,2340,en_33873108_33873277_36953117_1
_1_1_1,00.html Accessed on December 3, 2006

11. Available at: http://www.canhealth.com/News492.html Accessed on
December 7, 2006

12. Available at: http://www.nhinwatch.com/news.cms?newsId=1787
Accessed on December 7, 2006

13. Available at: http://www.omnimedix.org/news_pr2006-12-06.html Accessed
on December 7, 2006

Conclusion

Ours is a perpetually changing world, change that should evoke feelings of

pride in our ability to harness for the advancement of humanity. Put differently, it is change we should dare not so harness lest we have not even anything much more pride to spare. Thus, we must see the challenges imminent and remote, tackle, and overcome them in a determined effort to keep our health services working efficiently and cost-effectively, the key ingredients in any effort to achieve the dual healthcare delivery objectives we have so much talked about in this e-book. On the one hand, it seems quite idyllic that we have made so much progress as humans, not just in understanding and treating diseases, but also in identifying the potential for life hidden in us all, which we could deploy in our quest for health and wellness. One such potential is that of taking control of our life and what we do with, whether to exercise or not to, or to smoke or not to, or indulge in any other lifestyle that could make the difference to how long and healthy we live, for example. This is not to mention the chemicals in nature that could assist us in so doing, of which many of us are aware, anti-oxidants, for example, although the extent to which we shun or embrace them is another matter. This is also the case with the technologies, healthcare information and communication technologies, that is, which could help us, achieve the dual healthcare delivery goals, but we still also in the main, essentially shun.

The point here, and this has been the enduring theme of this e-book, that it is

time we took a different outlook to matters pertaining to our health, accept the inevitability of change and the need to adapt to it, all the time, ensuring that we are able to deliver qualitative health services to all, efficiently and cost-effectively. The link between health and the other sectors of the economy of any society is so basic that to do otherwise would be courting trouble, literally, which is not just in the interest of the populace, but also of the country's overall economic growth and sustainable development. There is indeed no intuitive sense in not pursuing these noble dual healthcare delivery objectives, as in the end, they are the engine so to say that drive life and society, and our world, and whichever way we look at it, and from which country, or health system we are, nothing perhaps holds truer. The choice then is ours.